# About the Author

Nicola Smuts-Allsop is a consulting astrologer living in the United Kingdom. Originally from South Africa, she completed her first studies at the Rod Suskin School of Astrology in Cape Town, and completed a Diploma in Medieval Astrology with AstroLogos in the UK. Nicola has recently graduated from Canterbury Christ Church University, with a Master's Degree in Myth, Cosmology and The Sacred.

Nicola has specialised in this field and has undergone fertility treatment herself. She is a mother of two adult children and can empathise and understand the pain and the desperation of trying to conceive. She lectures internationally on her fertility work and her research and methods in this field are pioneering and unique. Her success in diagnosing fertility issues in charts and finding potentially fertile times to try In Vitro Fertilisation (IVF) and other reproductive treatments has been published in *The Sunday Times* (London), *The London Times*, and *The Daily Mail*. Her work has also been featured on national television (*Free Spirit, Top Billing*) in South Africa.

You can find out more through Nicola's website
www.fertilityastrology.com

# FERTILITY ASTROLOGY
*A Modern Medieval Textbook*

NICOLA SMUTS-ALLSOP

The Wessex Astrologer

Published in 2018 by
The Wessex Astrologer Ltd
4A Woodside Road
Bournemouth
BH5 2AZ

For a full list of our titles go to www.wessexastrologer.com

© Nicola Smuts-Allsop 2018

Nicola Smuts-Allsop asserts the moral right to be recognised as the author of this work

Cover Design by Jonathan Taylor

A catalogue record for this book is available at The British Library

ISBN 9781910531259

The information contained in this book is for interest only and does not constitute medical advice.

No part of this book may be reproduced or used in any form or by any means without the written permission of the publisher. A reviewer may quote brief passages.

# Contents

Foreword
*Rod Suskin* vii

Preface
*How to read this book* ix

1
*What is Fertility Astrology?* 1

2
*Narrative Medicine and Fertility Myths* 9

3
*Case Study: Amanda* 24

4
*Case Study: Nancy and Lisa* 49

5
*Case Study: Raylene and Jacques* 74

6
*Brief Case Studies* 99

7
*Methods in Review* 113

8
*Signatures of Fertility* 129

9
*A Concluding Parable* 160

Appendix
*Almuten Worksheet* 163

Glossary 165

Bibliography 171

Dedication

This book is dedicated to all the women who have struggled with infertility – and those who still are.

# Acknowledgements

This book has had many midwives, but its conception (apologies) must be credited to Dr. Bernadette Brady, who, on a visit to South Africa to speak at a conference I was hosting, rearranged my brain and my study and instructed me on how to begin writing it. I was introduced to the marvellous Ysha de Donna who so generously allowed me to express myself without judgment. A first draft appeared on the horizon, and then I took time off to study a master's degree at Canterbury.

The hugely talented Dr. Jenn Zahrt took over as a more critical, academic editor and a more serious draft formed. The last trimester saw the final touches by Margaret Cahill, my publisher, who tweaked and packaged my work into what you have in your hand. The artist who painted the picture featured on the cover, Tracy Payne, is a childhood friend. I discovered the painting while on holiday in South Africa, and to my delight, she had painted the word NOW over the ancient figures of Shiva and Parvati, mirroring my integration of medieval traditional astrology and modern medical treatment.

During the final preparation of the book I had the good fortune to work with Wade Caves on the chart wheel design; I really appreciated both the clean, clear lines of his charts, and his support for the book and my astrology. When I was first learning astrology, medieval or traditional techniques – indeed the very texts themselves – were extremely hard to come by, and the internet was but a foetus….(think dial-up modems!) So the younger set (of which Wade is one) have been fortunate to have had access to newly published works from older sources, and consequently there is a shift towards more rigorous astrology. There is also a shift towards 'whole sky' astrology, using the fixed stars, and I have drawn heavily on the work of Bernadette Brady to give my predictions a broader context and a deeper interpretation.

I would like to acknowledge the life work of Robert Hand (also Robert Schmidt and Robert Zoller) and the Project Hindsight translations, without which my astrological technique would be very much poorer.

It would be remiss of me not to mention my very dear friend and colleague Rod Suskin, who not only taught me astrology, but who has patiently heard every idea or thought that contributed to this book. I was an unruly student, and my thoughts are not exactly linear, so his continued friendship is terribly precious to me.

Lastly… I really need to thank Himself, who has put up with 'this astrology business' and who never complains about the time I spend away from the family, either holed up in my study or travelling to another conference.

Nicola Smuts-Allsop
Bath
March 2018

# Foreword

## Rod Suskin

Most astrologers are familiar with the connections between astrology and mythology – both those myths that predate the astrology we know and those that we looked to later to help explain what we saw in the stars. As much as mythology helps us understand ourselves, it is rare to find a close marriage between astrological technique and mythological narrative that produces a direct, practical application of narrative healing. That can be found in this book.

Nicola's astrology is revolutionary for many reasons. One is quite simply that she takes deeply classical methods such as the Almuten of pregnancy and directs it, an unprecedented use of almutens yet revelatory in its results. Another is that she brings her astrology into the contemporary health paradigms of narrative medicine and shows that astrology fits into these new paradigms and ways of understanding ourselves just as it did in ancient times and throughout the ages, without having to alter the astrology to fit the modern paradigm.

This is a significant point. Nicola does not require us to alter or abandon the astrology we know, which has been used throughout our history; nor does her innovation mean we have to accept a paradigm of astrology distant from those we already know.

She reminds us that fertility itself is not a subject new to astrology, but the results of using many of the largely symbolic traditional methods common today have been found wanting at best. Difficulty conceiving is a prevalent issue and one which causes much anxiety, and methods such as IVF, which are often resorted to, in themselves prolong anxiety through expense and discomfort.

Since there are so few alternative options, it is not surprising that many specialists in the field of fertility have been open to Nicola's work in an effort to minimise the challenges for these patients. This has enabled her to help people who might otherwise have never consulted an astrologer, as well as encourage professionals in other fields such as medicine to see the value of astrology, and indeed astrology itself in an altogether new light.

The same will happen to you when you apply the methods in this book. While Nicola does not fall into the thorny trap of attempting to prove her work using the limitations of empirical methods, her work with doctors and the many successful results people have had with her methods speak to a new paradigm in which to measure astrological results. Nicola suggests that astrology *is* a narrative healing method, and thus allows the reader to contemplate and experiment with the use of her clear methodology to help resolve other challenges our clients face.

I have witnessed Nicola's progress through the vast knowledge network of astrology since its very beginning, and it is inspiring – and sometimes mind-boggling – to see where her penetrating, enquiring intellect has taken her without ever steering her away from her solid roots in traditional and contemporary methods.

I know that what awaits you, the reader, is a journey that will challenge, stretch and grow your astrology too.

Rod Suskin
Cape Town
January 2018

# How to read this book

This is a thoroughly contemporary book of medieval astrology, which may well present you with new techniques and also some that may seem to contradict what you already know. I use major case studies that demonstrate by example how to read charts for fertility questions; each and every story is unique, and each time I interpret a chart the results are slightly different from the client before. And while the departure point for all the delineations is based in the medieval tradition of astrology, the modern techniques you are more familiar with can come to play a role as the delineation proceeds. Despite the variances of how my methods are employed between cases, a consistent theme runs throughout the narratives.

Also know that there is no 'definitive' method of interpreting someone's fertile potential; signatures can only go so far. As you will find, the actual signatures vary slightly from case to case, and my interpretations reflect the specific nature of each chart and situation. You can read these case studies as if you were reading a story, and let the historical and technical information dispersed throughout sink in and take root. As you begin to work with clients you will hone a similar adaptability in your practice that I demonstrate in the following pages.

In addition, although I work globally, most of my research is based on charts from South Africa (and to a lesser extent, the United Kingdom), and as such it will have a cultural bias you may not be familiar with. However, the diversity of my client base has allowed me to glean an understanding of fertility that transcends racial and cultural boundaries, and so I am able to understand the core issues that affect women more broadly. It's worth keeping this in mind as you read.

I hope that this book will teach you the nuances of navigating fertile potentials through the stories of brave couples whose infertility confounded the medical profession. Each of the people in the case studies I present worked with astrological advice to overcome the obstacles that stood between them and parenthood. Let's get pregnant!

# 1

## What is Fertility Astrology?

Astrology is, in essence, the means by which we are able to measure the quality of a given moment in time and to see growth cycles begin and mature. In agriculture the tradition of planting seeds on a waxing moon according to farmer's almanacs is a deeply ingrained ritualisation of planting according to time and season. Yet in modern society we find it hard to take the next logical step and apply this tenet to all life – including human life.

In tribal cultures a good crop meant pregnant women, and pregnant women indicated a good crop. It seemed to the locals that if the women in the tribe were fecund, then the environment was viable for agricultural success and an increase in livestock. Communities would plant according to the rising of certain constellations, and these constellations were (and still are) seasonal – stars rise and set in more or less the same place in the sky for each location, year in and year out. So began the rhythm of life in certain latitudes all over the world. Why do our modern medical professionals refuse to use, or even make themselves aware of these rising and setting constellations as indicators of fertility for their patients? Do we, as a society, honestly believe that the seasonal changes, the ancient dialogue our forefathers had with the stars, is suddenly defunct, obsolete in our globalised and technological age? Why do we assume that one technology makes another one redundant? Should we not be using every technique at our disposal, considering the enormity of the fertility problems facing the human race?

I ask these questions because astrology is so easy to use. It does not require medical intervention. It does not require a religious conversion. Considering its usefulness, it is practically free. Put most simply, fertility astrology is twofold: descriptive and predictive. In its descriptive form, fertility astrology helps us arrive at diagnoses for infertility when current medical science has lost hope. In its predictive form, fertility astrology is a description of the quality of time during which a client would like to try to conceive and a judgement on the likelihood of success. In my experience working with clients, I have found that each person has roughly 2.5 lucky times a year. If one were to be speculating (either with money or with wanting to conceive), it would make sense to use these fortunate times to undertake projects which require a little extra luck.

## Turning to medieval astrology

Many of the techniques I present in this book are rooted in medieval astrology, so it is imperative to review the medieval astrological mindset because it differs significantly from modern practices of astrology. Robert Zoller, in a lecture he gave to the Astrological Lodge of London, suggested that modern astrologers, particularly psychological astrologers, have limited their ability to predict using medieval techniques since they do not practise their astrology using a medieval frame of mind.[1] He asserted that modern astrologers put the native at the centre of the chart so that each and every house is seen as affecting them personally – every transit is something that will happen directly to them. This very personalised, egocentric way of approaching the chart leads the client to expect to feel every transit and have every interpretation happen to *them*, directly. When nothing of significance happens to them, modern clients criticise astrology saying that, in the absence of any perceived manifestation, astrology doesn't work. Zoller contrasts this approach with the medieval astrological viewpoint, which

> limits the native to the 1st house and to the ruler of the 1st house and qualifies the native in terms of the planets aspecting the 1st house. All the other houses are circumstantial, i.e. they stand *around* the native… such a planet may relate to *someone or something else*. So that you can use the rules of prediction to determine whether you are going to be affected by *someone else* or not. This discrimination of self and other is essential if one is to have any chance of determining who will be the recipient of any configuration affecting the natal figure.[2]

Similarly, if we approach fertility astrology with a modern lens we run into problems of the same nature.

For instance, modern nations regulate the fertility industry with laws governing the treatments, the clinics, and a patient's constitutional rights. Many of us live in democracies that lead us to believe that we are all born equal and that all things apply equally to each of us. So, against the background of equal opportunity and access to treatment for fertility, we believe that we should all be able to get pregnant if and when we like. But astrologically, we know that not all charts are equal. Siblings are a testament to this simple truth: one child, born into the same family, in the same circumstances, and with the same opportunity for learning, nurturing and nourishment, has the potential to achieve a greatness perhaps denied to her siblings – as evidenced by her birth chart. Also, the conditions and contingencies that come in to influence the course of our lives will be different for each of us – by virtue of the 'someone or something else' that, while indicated in our birth chart, have nonetheless an independent existence from us, and thus a different, and *unequal*, effect on each of us. So why do we insist on treating birth charts as if all are equal, in all ways?

One's chart would have been seen as a means to transcend, not to seek comfort. Medieval astrologers, frequently only employed by aristocracy, were concerned with death, plagues, pestilence, loss of fortune, and favour with the king.

The notion of equal opportunities for all has now led to modern governments passing legislation that parenthood is a constitutional right, and thus by implication an enforceable right. Try telling that to fertility specialists! They understand more than anyone that no amount of fertility treatment can guarantee a live birth. Yet it can be incredibly difficult to get pregnant. Research shows that there is only a 15 percent chance that a healthy couple in their twenties may conceive each month.[3] Only 15 percent! Where does that leave older women and couples with issues such as sperm morphology problems and hormonal imbalances? Where did that leave the medieval astrologer trying to predict a pregnancy for the king of Spain, without any modern medical knowledge of the condition of his sperm or his consort's eggs, and with no antibiotics to clear up any STIs that may be blocking her fallopian tubes?

Surprisingly, in the prediction of pregnancy, the medieval astrologer often succeeds where the modern astrologer fails. In modern astrology, the tools and sources that we have at our disposal to predict pregnancy are limited. Either too many points are used, or incomplete technique, or technique is applied incorrectly due to misunderstandings from translation or lumping together of methods. In the practice of medieval astrology, there is an understanding that one cannot predict anything that is not contained in the natal chart. A transit of Jupiter to the 11th house is not necessarily going to win someone the lottery, but in modern astrology such restraint is rarely practised in prediction.

In my predictive work in fertility astrology, I am based firmly in medieval technique, and I also utilise insight drawn from modern psychology – carefully – where it may serve the client's need. There is one shining opportunity for astrology to succeed where extremely talented and clever practitioners of modern medicine sometimes fail: and that is in the small but significant matter of timing. Astrology provides a unique suite of tools not available to these modern practitioners. In addition, by addressing the gap in timing, another gap is closed, that is, the fear and debilitating stress that often limit conception. With a proper knowledge of timing, this fear and stress are reduced and the chances of success increase dramatically. As a practising astrologer specialising in fertility issues for a decade, I can attest to astrology's efficacy in this field. This book seeks to provide a pathway through my methods to help you successfully assist your own clients in the journey to parenthood.

**Dispelling the myth of the 'Jonas Method'**

Before going into my timing techniques, I must emphasise what this book will not discuss and why. If one searches for fertility astrology on the internet, the most commonly occurring results cite the solar/lunar phase method proposed by a Slovakian doctor by the name of Dr Eugen Jonas. Jonas theorizes that a woman is most fertile whenever the Sun and Moon are in the same lunar phase relationship as in the natal chart. For example, if one is born with a natal balsamic Moon, then each time the Sun and Moon are in a balsamic relationship that is when the woman is most likely to conceive. In addition to proposing the proper window of fertility, his method accounted for the determination of biological sex as well. If conception occurred when the Moon was in a feminine sign, Jonas predicted a female child and if the Moon was in a masculine sign, a male child.[4] If only it were that easy!

Unfortunately, it isn't that easy. A brief examination of Jonas's research presents a number of problems that must be cleared up. First, his data fails to conform to acceptable scientific standards. He asked couples to report when they had sex, rather than creating scenarios for laboratory monitoring of them having sex. This is problematic because couples routinely fictionalise the conception of children to fit a more romantic narrative. For example, many people are averse to admitting that conception may have happened during drunken make-up sex, so these client reports suffer from the same kind of unreliability as eye-witness testimony. On this level, his research is unusable scientifically.

Second, no one has ever been able to reliably predict when conception actually happens. Medically speaking, there is a six-day window between the fertilisation of the egg and the implantation of the embryo in the uterus. This temporal gap puts Jonas's theory about the sign of the Moon predicting the sex of the embryo into question because, as should be clear to astrologers, the Moon moves substantially during this six-day window. Given this uncertainty it is therefore impossible to link the lunar phase with conception with any degree of accuracy, let alone predict the sex of the child. To account for this he asserts that the sign of the Moon during the woman's phase return determines the sex. But that is still too fuzzy. Which is it?

While Jonas's theory appears astrologically elegant, it has been proven to be of little practical use, especially since using techniques that rely on an implantation within a twenty-four hour window cannot be accommodated in most medical centres. Even if the lunar phase theory were to be proven accurate, it would still be impractical to use in the treatment of fertility. Such critical timing (such as twenty-four hour window) is far too stressful for patients to deal with. They are not in control of the operating theatres and adding to their distress is not helpful.

A final, and important, comment on this theory is that it appears to suggest that a woman is fertile not once but twice a month, each and every month. This has also been demonstrated to be an incorrect assumption. Most women, at some point in their fertile lives will not ovulate during their cycle due to stress or other factors, and most women's cycles are out of sync with their lunar phase relationship (meaning that they might be menstruating at the time of this lunar phase, or not ovulating). The statistic that women have a 15-percent chance of falling pregnant suggests that couples have roughly three fertile windows in a particular year.[5] In my practical and astrological experience, this correlates more accurately with the frequency of Jupiter forming aspects to their natal Sun, Moon or Ascendant, and the 'Almuten of Pregnancy', an astrological concept I introduce in this book. As will be seen in the pages that follow, if you are predicting potentially fertile times, you will have a greater time-frame to work with if you use the transits of Jupiter, a slow moving planet, rather than the Moon, the fastest planet. Using Jupiter as a timing planet makes scheduling embryo transfers less stressful, even if one has the support of a medical team. As I demonstrate, accurate prediction of pregnancy depends on more precise techniques than those popularised by Dr. Jonas in the twentieth century.

## A few more considerations

I have some further advice for astrologers who would like to specialise in the field of in/fertility. While I employ a great many medieval techniques in my astrology, I don't apply every one of them to every chart. For example, I do not delineate the preventional or conjunctional new Moon in every chart, as this is a general commentary and in my experience has little to do with in/fertility in the chart in particular. Similarly, while it could be useful to calculate the Alcocoden for each and every client, it is a technique that I seldom use, as it doesn't significantly add to the outcome of the consultation.

This book is written to introduce you to a new suite of astrological techniques to add to your current skill set. By all means take onboard the ideas in this text, but continue to further develop your own techniques concerning in/fertility. Ownership of technique is very important, as it builds confidence, and as we see in the following chapters, it is vital to the successful outcome of the consultation that the astrologer exercises consistent command of their techniques and delivers interpretations with authority. To do this requires experimentation with the techniques until you are able to generate some 'meaning response' with your clients. In other words: read, listen, and experiment until you are familiar with how you, as the astrologer, would like to approach the subject of in/fertility with your clients.

Note that very often your client will already be traumatised by the time they come to see you. They will have had the bad news that it is going to be very difficult for them to become parents. In many cases, their dreams and aspirations will have been destroyed, and they will probably be on some hormonal medication at the time, so expect an emotionally charged and intense session. Be aware that the first thing you will have to deal with is grief, the loss of a 'normal' narrative. First and foremost and the question hanging in the air is, 'What did I do to deserve this?' You, as the astrologer, need to have the skills to hold that pain while simultaneously providing hope, and keeping the client from falling apart. For married couples who come to see me, I sometimes begin by remarking on the wonderful relationship synastry of their charts, thereby supporting their marriage/partnership and consolidating them as a team. I might use humour in gentle teasing about emotional rollercoaster rides due to the drug regime the woman might be on. Often the partner of the client who sought me out is brought into the consultation reluctantly, and they need to be included right from the start in a matter-of-fact way, helping them to understand that this 'New Age astrology lark' is actually quite normal (and in my case, not even New Age).

It is important to say your client's name more than once, and remember if you're on Skype to look directly into the camera from time to time, so as to establish eye contact. I prefer to wear contact lenses for Skype consultations so that my glasses don't obscure my eyes while glancing at my notes or the screen. In the absence of other opportunities for therapeutic contact, such as touching their arm, you need to create as many ways as possible of connecting with your client.

Furthermore, it is vital to read some sort of disclaimer at the beginning of the session so that your clients are clear about the limits of astrology and your limitations as a practitioner. For instance, I make my clients nod or say 'yes' to the statement: 'you do know I am not a medical doctor, right?' And I never, ever, prescribe medications, herbs, or treatments without saying, 'please check with your medical doctor first'. Even if you strongly disagree with the medical treatment they are receiving, you need to support them and not undermine what their doctor has prescribed. You are not in a position to know all the facts and you're not being paid for such advice, even if you happen to be a medical fertility specialist. They need you to support them on their path, not to confuse them with contradictory advice.

Your main focus is to ascertain the reasons why they are not falling pregnant, determine whether these are psychological or physical, and, through dialogue, find a treatment plan for them and address the issue of the timing of whatever treatment they have chosen to use. Equally important is that they understand that astrology is not a miracle panacea that is going to fix physical issues such as chromosomal defects of egg or sperm, or a compromised uterus. By providing a clear framework of how astrology can help maximise their chances, you are managing their expectations and not compounding their disappointments.

While I'm happy to consult on reasons for infertility, and optimal times for attempting conception, I strictly avoid predicting biological sex. Sex discrimination is sometimes critical (especially in cases of hereditary diseases such as haemophilia, etc.), and the astrology we have at our disposal is just not accurate enough for me to feel comfortable taking that level of responsibility, never mind the other kinds of discrimination around social/cultural preference.

Finally, it should go without saying that you should keep your own judgements about your client's potential parenting skills or abilities in check. There is no telling who will be a brilliant or bad parent, and it's not your responsibility to decide whether or not someone is going to be good enough. People have criticised me in the past for 'adding to the world population problem', and, while it seems as though I am successful, I cannot possibly impact on this particular ecological issue if I tried. I help anyone: LGBTQI+, married, single mothers, surrogate mothers, and any religious persuasion under the Sun. When the clients contact me, I consult them. The rest is up to them. In the next chapter we will discuss some techniques for framing your work with your clients in an engaging and effective manner using narrative medicine and fertility myths.

**Notes**
1. Robert Zoller, lecture to the Astrological Lodge of London, Gloucester Place, London, UK (7 April 1997).
2. Italics mine.
3. Winston, Robert. *Infertility: A Sympathetic Approach*.
4. His teachings are presented in Ostrander, Sheila and Schroeder, Lynn, *Astrological Birth Control*.
5. *Infertility: A Sympathetic Approach*.

## 2

## Narrative Medicine and Fertility Myths

Fertility astrology is a subset of medical astrology, and 'the main function of medical astrology', according to Dr. Jane Ridder-Patrick, 'is *not* to provide an orthodox medical diagnosis, but an astro-somatic one which elicits meaning and points to root causes'.[6] The concept of *eliciting* meaning has taken on a new life in the contemporary practice of medicine.

**Narrative Medicine**

In the late 1990s Dr. Rita Charon pioneered a new branch of medicine focused on the power of narratives in the practice of modern medicine. After spending her early career as an MD, she went back to graduate school and obtained a PhD in English, and applied what she learned to the clinical setting. She now directs the Program in Narrative Medicine at Columbia University in New York City. In her book, *Narrative Medicine*, Charon says that in the course of her medical practice:

> I came to understand that what my patients paid me to do was to listen expectantly and attentively to extraordinarily complicated narratives – told in words, gestures, silences, tracings, images, laboratory test results, and changes in the body – and to cohere all these stories into something that made provisional sense, enough sense, that is, on which to act.[7]

When Charon discusses her first encounter with narrative and medicine, she reveals a story she constructed about a patient she had once seen briefly – a hypothesis about what was going on with the patient. Later, when seeing the patient again, Dr. Charon asked about the actual situation the patient had been going through, and the patient shared a deeper story that did not match the one that Charon had imagined in her mind. Charon said her 'hypothesis acted like a prosthetic device or a tool with which to get to the truth'.[8] This encounter served to show Charon her own bias and how that impeded her ability to see what was really going on with her patient:

> The price for a technologically sophisticated medicine seems to be impersonal, calculating treatment from revolving sets of specialists who, because they are consumed with the scientific elements in health care, seem divided from the ordinary human experiences that surround pain, suffering and dying.[9]

What we learn from this is that even fictional explanatory narratives have their place in healing. There is no concept of one truth, but rather an external prompt in order to trigger or animate the soul to move in a particular direction.

Astrology is also just such a narrative tool. The natal chart is an external mechanism that creates a kind of objectivity. However, we run the risk of committing the same error of Charon's first (wrong) hypothesis when we rely too heavily on the technical (the chart, the signatures) instead of listening to the lived reality of our clients. As Charon shows in her work, interpretation is a constant factor in medical analysis.[10] She argues for a recognition of interpretational events outside the raw medical data in the interaction between patient and doctor and what is both said and unsaid. Seen this way, adding sensitive astrological interpretation back into the matrix of medical care can enhance the efficacy of the medicine.

According to Charon, the conflict of meaning centres around 'the singularity of the patient's life'.[11] She calls for medical practitioners to recognize the 'singular contexts that donate meaning to each clinical situation'.[12] Medical astrology already developed such a practice hundreds of years ago in the form of the decumbiture chart, or the chart for when the patient first falls ill. In the wake of the scientific revolution and our efforts to modernise medicine, we have forgotten a narrative system already developed for this singularity, both of the condition of sickness (decumbiture chart) and the patient (natal chart). Medical science reduces people to statistics and tick boxes. Astrology is unique to the patient so the diagnosis is made from a unique standpoint, not a generalised model. Charon points out a strong link between a patient's cosmology and their belief about the cause of disease. She says:

Even if, in retrospect, the hypothesis of causality is wrong... the hypothesis has functioned to limit uncertainty temporarily, giving at least the impression of purposeful action in the face of the disease and some help in tolerating the uncertainty that remains.[13]

This is a common phenomena, and one that is regularly used to demonstrate the 'flakiness' of alternative healing practices, which sometimes strain to fulfil scientific criteria in trials. Ben Goldacre says that, in fact, what most people are looking for is a diagnosis and any one will do, even a fictional one, which is what Charon also suggests. He states:

...alternative therapists don't just give placebo treatments; they also give what we might call 'placebo explanations' or 'placebo diagnoses': ungrounded, unevidenced, often fantastical assertions about the nature of the patient's disease, involving magical properties, or energy, or supposed vitamin deficiencies, or 'imbalances', which the therapist claims uniquely to understand.

And, here it seems that this 'placebo' explanation – even if grounded in sheer fantasy – can be beneficial to a patient.[14]

Take, for example, the diagnosis of endometriosis, which is a condition where fibroids form in the uterus, and uterine tissue grows outside of the uterus, sometimes strangling the fallopian tubes and enveloping the ovary. In the treatment of endometriosis, doctors are very eager to remove small polyps with laparoscopic surgery, as this is perceived by the patient to be finding and locating 'the problem' and the successful removal of 'the problem', resulting in a healthy uterus, ready for implantation and conception. Doctors are aware that there are many women who have such polyps and fibroids who successfully achieve pregnancy without intervention, and they also acknowledge that the scanning equipment is now so advanced that this is an opportunity to exercise an easy and effective 'placebo surgery', while simultaneously upholding medical ethical practice.

In a similar way, astrologers like to identify a 'problem transit' or planet, and once they find out which time cycle is causing difficulty, they are able at the very least to tell the client when that particularly difficult period is over, and when a more fortunate time is coming in the future. Such reassurances fit neatly into this model as defined by Charon and others.

Charon's main thesis boils down to the idea that one has to know how to read closely – how to understand and navigate narrative – in order to know how to treat a patient properly. Scientific medical evaluation is not enough, we need the precision of close reading as taught by the humanities too. When reading a poem it is the interpretation and the meaning found by the reader and the author that stimulate the imagination. The astrologer and the client likewise co-create the healing outcome.

**Listening**
When gathering information from a patient, Charon stresses the need to be fully present and listening to the person speaking.[15] Many doctors are often not looking directly at the patient and hearing what they say. Their heads are bowed down to the page and their hands are busy writing real-time what is being said out loud to them. This is entirely backwards. For Charon, the act of listening – really listening – to what the patient is saying allows for the establishment of a deeper connection. This lets the patient's story emerge without immediately subjecting it to interpretation because of the habits of shorthand notes. She recommends using the patient's own words. Quoting Sir Richard Bayliss, the former dean of Westminister Hospital Medical School, she says, 'Histories must be received, not taken'. This receptivity is what shifts the encounter, and, I suggest, moves it closer to becoming a situation of genuine healing. Here's how she does it:

> When I met patient X, I was using for the first time the new approach I invented for meeting a new patient. It begins simply with the invitation to 'tell me what you think I should know about your situation', and is followed by a commitment to listen and not – at least at the start – to write or even speak… It was only when I was able to forgo the ordering imperative (of compulsive note taking) that I became able to absorb what patients tell me without deranging their narratives into my own form of story. I listen as hard as I can – not taking notes during this part of the interview, not interrupting unless critical, not indicating one way or another what I consider salient or meaningful or interesting. *I try my best to register the dictation, the form, the images, the pace of speech. I pay attention* – as I sit there at the edge of my seat, absorbing what is being given – *to metaphors, idioms,*

*accompanying gestures, as well as plot and characters represented for me by the patient.*[16]

Charon is describing above how she elicits 'meaning' from the non-verbal communication from the patient.[17] Just as the creation and decoding of meaning is not limited to words alone, these seemingly insignificant gestures, or cultural expressions or archetypal identifications are just as important to Charon as the physical symptom. The recognition of these expressions of soul is the key to healing. She seeks the pivotal moment in the consultation where the breakthrough happens, where the patient is revealed as a whole person, a soul with a broken body, not just a body with broken parts. She anticipates the moment of interchange where the patient also acknowledges that they have been 'seen' for the first time, and when a recognition or transference takes place. She recognises that this space holds the potential for healing.

In his book *The Moment of Astrology*, Geoffrey Cornelius describes the moment when, in an astrological consultation, the energy (for want of a better word) changes, the client registers the 'truth' in the statement uttered by the astrologer and the astrologer recognises the signature as both apt and true. Together the client and astrologer make the meaningful connection to the problem or issue at hand. This recognition of the chart being radical, is the katarchic shift, when the primary cause of the issue is revealed and the consultation really begins. Cornelius elaborates on the meaning of katarche:

> Let us look at the non-astrological meanings of the term. The word carries several meanings depending on the context. The most general of these is 'beginning'. It may also refer to 'primacy, sovereignty, and basis'; 'the part of the sacrificial victim first offered'; and 'to begin the rites of sacrifice'. This last usage appears to be the most ancient, dating back to Homer.[18]

Thus, as I interpret it, Charon focuses on the moment when the soul or the spirit speaks. She waits for the revelation of the whole person, aside from the corporeal being in front of her. This to me relates nearly directly with that radical moment that Cornelius refers to when 'spirit' or 'the Gods' speak in the chart.[19]

We must meet the client half way, let them give us their gift, so that we may serve them properly. Knowing the tools of astrology gives us a certain power, certainly, but we are not all-knowing, and sometimes our vast knowledge can be a stumbling block if we are not open to the soul of the client in our midst. Charon states, 'like lawyers, teachers, historians, and journalists, healthcare professionals have come to realize... ethical demands of telling one's story and receiving the stories of others'.[20] Astrology accounts for all those factors, especially with the time-bound nature of pregnancy. In the words of Tvetzen Todorov, a Russian narratologist, 'meaning does not exist before being articulated and perceived'.[21] Charon adds: 'the telling does not merely expose or report that which exists prior to the narrating. *It produces it*'.[22] The patient is creating themselves in the consultation room, and we are creating alongside them as we take part in the conversation and build the narrative together with them. Meaning and response are inextricably bound up in one another.

In the practice of astrology – a narrative language of symbol and archetype needing interpretation and participation with the client, and which employs the imagination and indeed 'suspension of belief' in some cases – the possibility that astrology is functioning as an inert placebo cannot be dismissed. I am not suggesting that astrologers lie, or that astrology is fake or that we are not affected physically by the planets, but I do want to suggest that if we do want to be accepted into a dialogue with the medical profession, we might have to repackage our astrology to include the idea that we deal in (and heal with!) 'meaning responses'.

Causal explanations for astrology's efficacy evade us still. And until there is some conclusive study demonstrating a measurable (read: physical) causal effect – the only type of evidence that science seems to allow as real – we will be more successful by focusing on the direct causes that astrology, as a narrative tradition, does have: we converse with our clients about themselves using a tradition of stories related to the astrological data, the client's birth data or time of questioning us, and the rest of the human experience that comes into the discussion. Language and what happens in the consultation with the client cause direct shifts in understanding. The 'meaning response' angle, as I have shown through this discussion of placebo, is far more persuasive than investigating planetary rays or some other physical causal relation between humans on earth and the stars. The fact is, the moment of astrology consists of the astrologer generating a specific type of narrative with the client.

In the popular imagination surrounding astrology, the search for a physical causal explanation for its effects still persists. The public, including our clients, often wish to cling to the romantic notion that, like the tides, we humans are all affected by the Moon. And I would suggest that if your client is desiring that kind of 'enchantment' narrative, then you should let that suspension of belief do just that. The consultation room is packed with all sorts of contradictions, and variable truths. One more contradiction is not going to make the outcome less truthful or less meaningful for the client. What cannot be overlooked is the other direct causal effects of astrology: the conversation in the consultation room.

Indeed Cheryl Mattingly refers directly to fiction and fantasy as being the cause of healing when she states that "healing dramas open up a world of possibilities, allowing participants to inhabit 'as if' worlds that have transformative, sometimes even socially radical, implications for becoming".[23] Charon similarly believes in 'the redemptive force of narrative to heal'.[24] Now I would like to explore one of many deep cultural narratives that inform astrological practice. Hopefully after reading this and other myths in the context of fertility astrology you will see them in a new light.

## Inanna – An Originary Fertility Myth

While there are many myths about fertility throughout various cultures, in this chapter I discuss a prominent myth that has revealed itself in my practice, with its ancestral beliefs about fertility, timing, and the interrelationship between stellar imagery and cultural practice: the myth of Inanna. This ancient Sumerian myth offers a multi-layered exploration of the rites of passage of life and death, while simultaneously telling the story of the rising and setting of the planet Venus. The interpretative valence of this myth speaks to many disciplines.[25] I interpret this myth on three levels. Firstly, the myth functions as a template for therapists and healers that illuminates the nature of human crisis and how we heal. Secondly, in the context of the astrological cycle of Venus, I link the myth to the understanding that astrologers have about Venus and how they interpret Venus in the astrological chart. Finally, I highlight the relevance of this myth in the world of fertility. Before proceeding along these lines, we must examine the narrative of the myth itself.

The myth of Inanna begins with Inanna's trip to the underworld to see her sister Ereshkigal, whose husband Gugulanna (Bull of Heaven) has died, and to attend the funeral rites. Inanna is well aware of the dangers of approaching the underworld and appeals to her maidservant, Ninshubur, to send for help in the event that she does not return. On her journey, Inanna must approach the seven gates to the abode of Ereshkigal, and, at each of these gates, she must disrobe and leave behind a component of her material wealth – her crown, her jewellery, her clothing – until she is finally completely naked, no symbols of authority, no symbols of social status or wealth, no badges of femininity.

At this point Inanna is somewhat frightened of Ereshkigal; she has already alerted her maidservant to the possibility that some harm might come to her. In some interpretations of the myth, Inanna is haughty and proud and wears her garments as talismans of power.[26] She is aware of her charisma and is thus humiliated to be stripped off her raiments at the gates. However, she also intends to return to the light, as she leaves behind her precious possessions including her crown and other assets that define her as queen of her world.

Ereshkigal is likened to Kali, or Lilith, the angry ruthless destroyer. She is jealous of Inanna – who lives in the light, and who has recently married. It is thought that Ereshkigal is the psychological shadow of Inanna, the darker side of femininity within all women, passionate and yet destructive, warrior-like and yet crippled by emotional pain.[27] As Inanna reaches her sister in the underworld, Ereshkigal finds it impossible to allow herself to receive the beautiful Innana, whose husband is still waiting for her in the light. Inanna represents the natural fecundity and fertility of women, the natural grace of a queen and the agricultural skills of husbandry and commerce.[28] Ereshkigal has none of these gifts. She remains barren, but in constant pain. She has no generosity as she has nothing to give. In fact, I argue that her gift is the destruction of stasis, so that something else can be reborn. So when Inanna enters the underworld, Ereshkigal, in a fit of rage, fixes Inanna with a stare of death. Inanna withers, and her corpse is hung on a meat hook in the halls of Hades as a reminder of the destructive power of her jealous sister.

When Inanna doesn't return on time, Ninshubur goes to the God Enki who conjures the two figures Galatur and Kurgarra, who begin to search for Inanna. In some retellings these beings are little parasites, in others they are known as dirt from underneath Enki's fingernails.[29] These little beings are small enough to pass through the gates undetected. They approach Ereshkigal, who is still bereft and in mourning for her husband, and appeal to her by effectively echoing her mourning call, that is, by telling her 'we hear your pain' over and over again:

> The *kurgarra* and *galatur* heeded Enki's words. They set out for the underworld. Like flies, they slipped through the cracks of the gates. They entered the throne room of the Queen of the Underworld.
>
> No linen was spread on her body. Her breasts were uncovered. Her hair swirled around her head like leeks.
>
> Ereshkigal was moaning: 'Oh! Oh! My inside!'
> They moaned: 'Oh! Oh! Your inside!'
> She moaned: 'Ohhhh! My outside!'
> They moaned: 'Ohhhh! Your outside!'
> She groaned: 'Oh! Oh! My belly!'
> They moaned: 'Oh! Oh! Your belly!'
>
> [...]
>
> Ereshkigal stopped.
> She looked at them.
> She asked: 'Who are you,
> Moaning – groaning – sighing with me? If you are gods, I will bless you.
> If you are mortals, I will give you a gift.
> I will give you the water-gift, the river in its fullness.'
>
> The *kurgarra* and *galatur* answered: 'We do not wish it.'
> Ereshkigal said: 'I will give you the grain-gift, the fields in harvest.'
> The *kurgarra* and *galatur* said: 'We do not wish it.'
> Ereshkigal said: 'Speak then! What do you wish?'
> They answered: 'We wish only the corpse that hangs from the hook on the wall.'
> Ereshkigal said: 'The corpse belongs to Inanna.'
>
> They said:
> 'Whether it belongs to our queen, Whether it belongs to our king, That is what we wish.'

The corpse was given to them.

The *kurgarra* sprinkled the food of life on the corpse. The *galatur* sprinkled the water on the corpse.
Inanna arose…[30]

In their call and response echo of Ereshkigal's pain, they effectively mirror her own suffering back to herself and she feels acknowledged. By their compassionate and all embracing support, Ereshkigal is able to access that kind and loving connection and so, after a negotiation, she releases Inanna to them.

This type of mourning song finds resonance in an eighth-century religious practice: the Catholic Vespers. The word 'vesper' originates from the Latin for 'evening, the evening star'.[31] This can be compared to the Greek 'hesperos', which means 'evening, or west', where the planets and sun set along the horizon. Venus, appearing as an evening star, also shares this name 'vesper'. Being only visible at night, and, hence, the underworld, Ereshkigal is the mythological representative of the evening apparition of Venus; whereas Inanna is the apparition of the morning star Venus.[32]

The first line of the Catholic Vespers of the Office of the Dead reads 'placebo Domino in regione vivorum'.[33] The first word of this line, 'placebo', translates to 'I shall please'. In the myth, we witness Galatur and Kurgarra treating Ereshkigal to a type of Vesper. They sing to please her, and function as a placebo that releases her from her suffering and allows her, in turn, to release Inanna and to heal. Through this act, we find a potent suggestion of a connection between the ancient Sumerian myth and orthodox Catholic practice.

Returning now to the astrological Venus, the myth reveals the placebo, the mourning song, as the critical transition point between Venus as evening star, the suffering Ereshkigal, and Venus as morning star, Inanna reborn from the underworld.[34] The return of Inanna from the depths of the underworld depends upon this moment of compassionate recognition. In this way, the Sumerians embedded their associations of death and life and observations of the astronomical Venus into a primal myth. As Wolkenstein and Kramer note:

Ereshkigal, the neglected side of Inanna, has certain qualities that are similar to Lilith's. Both are connected to the night-time aspects of the feminine – the powerful, raging sexuality and the deep wounds accumulated from life's rejections – which seek solace in physical union only. Lilith usually flees from rejections; Ereshkigal withdraws 'underground'... The powerful Lilith of Inanna's adolescent days had to be sent away so Inanna's life-exploring talents could be developed. But now that Inanna has become Queen of her city, wife to her beloved, mother to her children, she is more able to face what she has neglected and feared: the instinctual, wounded, frightened part of herself. She now hears, and is capable of responding to, the labor call of Ereshkigal in the Great Below.[35]

There is a certain willingness on the part of Inanna to explore death and sacrifice; she is aware that there is a need to to visit the underworld – Kramer describes it as a 'calling'. He clarifies this by saying that the correct translation of the first line of *The Descent of Inanna* should read, 'From the Great Above she set her ear to the Great Below',[36] not her 'mind' as is commonly quoted. This is because Kramer believes that Inanna was constantly aware of the underworld and the necessity to be attentive to the call to go down there. It seems as if Inanna expects the call and responds to it. This also reminds the reader of the cyclical nature of things, Inanna has risen to the highest office – she is queen, she has authority, she has mastered the material world. Once achieving the high point of the cycle, there is a natural process of decline, decay or descent. This rise and fall has an astrological diurnal correlate. One can view this as a planet achieving the most elevated position of the Midheaven, with all the authority of the 10th house, and then the slow descent to the cardinal west point of the 7th house to set in darkness, past the midnight point of the nadir, and finally to rise again in the east, at the Ascendent. Inanna has achieved much in the material world and is recognising a need to address the spiritual. Her withdrawing to the underworld is her turning to her shadow persona, in the form of Ereshkigal, in order to redress an imbalance.

But Ereshkigal is not entirely evil. Silvia Perera links Ereshkigal to gestation and the transformative process of pregnancy itself.[37] She reframes it in a feminist way to acknowledge the breakdown of material and its reconstitution in another form. When Inanna emerges, she carries the wisdom of Ereshkigal's world in her. In its own way becoming pregnant is a descent into the underworld. A pregnant woman loses her singular identity. She often loses much else as well: her body morphs, her sexual drive shifts, her strength, health and mobility in the world experience extreme fluctuation. As Valerie Hartouni has shown, her behaviour and rights are often also restricted.[38] The woman must temporarily sacrifice herself, while new life forms in her own bodily underworld.

Although it seems as though Inanna sacrificed herself to the underworld, the real sacrifice comes when she is allowed to return to her rightful place in the world, but she has to replace herself with someone else. Beings who have been allowed to return from the underworld must send someone in their place to appease the death that has taken place. Inanna chooses to sacrifice her husband Dumuzi; in her judgement he did not mourn her properly and was too interested in his new-found power as king and his place in the world. His attitude is that he tended to her kingdom while she was away adventuring to the underworld. Her attitude is that he did not miss her enough or appreciate her allowing him to take her throne. Without going into too much detail on this section of the myth, what I want to highlight here is that a woman (Inanna) is leading a man (Dumuzi) into the underworld (the spiritual dimension).

This is useful to recognize for two reasons. First, in my fertility practice I am often stunned to notice how often a birth follows a death in the families that are trying to conceive. I proactively ask about the health of parents and older relatives and if someone close to the family (not always a blood relative) has passed away. I have observed that events of this nature are heightened at times of conception and that often a physical birth after grief and recognition of soul can take place. Second, it is usually the woman who leads the man (or partner) into the consultation room, but not after going there herself first. Many women feel as though they need to 'do' something more to get pregnant. They need to give up something: wine, coffee, gym, work, being independent. The list of things they are willing to sacrifice is long and detailed, and they are willing. They understand that something has to shift and sacrifice is needed. They draw their partners towards the spiritual path by insisting on seeing an astrologer, an acupuncturist, a healer, a shaman. They feel the need to address the spiritual as well as the physical. Modern medical practitioners can only offer mechanics, drugs, and technology. It is up to intuitive women to find the spiritual midwives, those who usher souls from the other side, those who can identify with pain and suffering. These women seek to find those healers who will come for them if they do not return from the underworld, and they seek those who can summon the Galatur and the Kurgarra to cry with them. These women who seek my help are often as angry as Ereshkigal, in her barrenness and her empty sexual rapaciousness; they are as angry as Lilith. Feelings of vengefulness and jealousy are only surface deep and triggered by a wrong word – such is the energy of the shadow of the fertile, Alpha female Inanna.

On the one hand, infertile clients want logical and reasoned explanations as to why they are not pregnant in spite of multiple treatments, and yet they also acknowledge that destiny might be playing a role. They try to understand their destiny, all the while trying to control it too, by offering sacrifices of money or charity or acts of contrition and supplication to whomever will give them relief and the baby they desire. As the myth of Inanna's descent shows us, this contradiction is human nature. It is who we are. We have to identify with both the Inanna and the Ereshkigal in all of us, and we have to yield to the compassion of the Kurgarra and Galatur and see our pain mirrored and honoured before we are allowed the release from our physical and spiritual stagnation.

The healing wisdom and power of the Inanna myth rests in the placebo, the mourning song of the Kurgarra and Galatur; and that is precisely where I locate the role of the astrologer in fertility work. As an astrologer, I take the position of being the Kurgarra and Galatur, not aligned to either sex, impartial but able to be compassionate, and yet on a mission to acknowledge the grief and to retrieve life in the situation. Through my communication with the client, I am able to mirror and hold space for pain until release is found. This often prepares the way for spiritual healing as well as physical healing and the ability of the patient to heal her/himself through identification with the shadow, and through acceptance and submission to the life force which courses through us all.

This life force is subject to seasons and changes in time, and it must be recognised that these cycles are different for each of us and we cannot all be in the underworld at the same time. Everyone takes a turn, and it is necessary for us to play a role in our fellow human's descent. We can be either the gatekeepers, removing possessions in order for others to descend, or we can be the carefree opportunistic king, making hay in the sunshine until our turn arrives. We can also be Enki, who has to fashion the Kurgarra and Galatur, in order to save our daughters, even though we might think they deserve their punishment. Or we can be the loyal faithful servant who has to call for help. Whichever role, there is a good chance that we are playing multiple parts in many plays in our lives and sometimes we are descending and sometimes we ascend. It is merely a function of seasons, a dance of planets, but in this human story, we all play a role.

The most powerful message in this myth is directly focused on the role of the astrologer.

The heroes in this story are the Kurgarra and Galatur; they manage to contain the pain that Ereshkigal is feeling, and they mirror it back to her in such a way as to allow her to feel compassion for herself, and then for others. Narratives create meaning, and they can transform.

From considerations of the use of narrative in medicine, as well as the myth of Inanna's descent to the underworld, we have a rich archive of mythological and historical material to accompany us into the client room. Now that we have covered this ground, we can turn to case studies. In these next few chapters, I will walk you through the methods and techniques needed to be able to use astrology to assist clients in understanding their fertile potential and achieving parenthood.

**Notes**

6. My emphasis. Ridder-Patrick, Jane. 'The Healing Power of Astrology', *The Astrological Journal* (July/August 2014): 11–15, 11.
7. Charon, Rita *Narrative Medicine: Honoring the Stories of Illness*, p.4.
8. Ibid, p.6.
9. Ibid.
10. Ibid p.26.
11. Ibid p.27.
12. Ibid.
13. Ibid p.28.
14. Goldacre, Ben. *Bad Science*, p.75.
15. *Narrative Medicine*, p.187.
16. Ibid. See also the chapter on Therapeutic placebo effects in Irving Kirsch, *The Emperor's New Drugs: Exploding the Antidepressant Myth*.
17. C.f., Moerman, D.E., Jonas, WB. 'Deconstructing the Placebo Effect and Finding the Meaning Response.' *Annals of Internal Medicine*. 136, pp.471-476.
18. Cornelius, Geoffrey. *The Moment of Astrology*, p.127.
19. Ibid p.29.

20. *Narrative Medicine* p.41.
21. Tvetzen Todorov, as cited in *Narrative Medicine*, p.61.
22. Ibid p. 45.
23. Mattingly, C. *The Paradox of Hope: Journeys Through a Clinical Borderland*.
24. *Narrative Medicine*, p.80.
25. Silvia Perera has examined it using a Jungian approach in her book *Descent to the Goddess: A Way of Initiation for Women*. The folklorist Diane Wolkenstein has dramatised its feminine aspects in her book with Samuel Noah Kramer, *Inanna: Queen of Heaven and Earth*. And, Samuel Noah Kramer, a cuneiformist, has focused on it as a historical document: Diane Wolkenstein, and Samuel Noah Kramer, *Sumerian Mythology*.
26. *Inanna: Queen of Heaven* p.56.
27. Ibid p.157–60.
28. *Descent to the Goddess* and *Inanna: Queen of Heaven*.
29. *Inanna: Queen of Heaven*, pp.64, 160.
30. These words are from the original translation by Kramer from the stone tablets in Cuniform. Ibid, pp.64–67.
31. Collins Dictionary. C14.
32. Personal communication with Bernadette Brady. Fixed Star workshop, 24 June 2003.
33. Psalm 114:9.
34. Some practising astrologers, such as Adam Gainsburg, make a distinction between the superior and inferior conjunctions of Venus in relation to this myth. I consider both periods of invisibility of the planet Venus to be resonant with the mythology of Inanna's descent. See Adam Gainsburg, *The Light of Venus*.
35. *Inanna: Queen of Heaven and Earth*, p.160.
36. Ibid, p.xvii.
37. *Descent to the Goddess*, p.24.
38. See Hartouni, Valerie. *Cultural Conceptions* p.41: 'In 1982,…a small group of obstetricians and geneticists declared that "medicine [was] far enough along for them to start treating foetuses as patients". With this declaration came the rapid expansion of efforts not only to treat the "foetal patient" but to protect it from potential abuse of neglect. Juvenile courts subsequently began to assume jurisdiction over the content of pregnant women's wombs and right-to-lifer efforts to reduce foetuses through forced medical intervention or incarceration of the women carrying them were intensified and highly publicised.

    Increasingly subject to legal scrutiny and criminal prosecution were pregnant women who smoke, drank, and had sex, ingested legal as well as illicit drugs, refused major surgery (e.g. caesareans), failed to follow the advice or instructions of their physicians, failed to obtain adequate prenatal care, worked or lived in proximity to teratogenic substances, or engaged in any range of activities deemed "reckless" and potentially detrimental to foetal life'.

# 3

# Case Study – Amanda

This case study is meant to be a practical guide through many of the delineation techniques I use in a consultation. The practice of fertility astrology weaves many strands of medieval and traditional technique together, and, given this complexity, it makes more sense to teach through example than through discussions of technique. Once you have gone through the elements that are key to a successful client session, you can go back and review the astrology you need more time with. Chapter Seven provides further reflection on the methods I use, but it is beneficial first to read through the following case studies in order, so you can see how I use these techniques in context. Without further ado, I would like to introduce you to Amanda.

Amanda and I met at a mutual friend's cocktail party. She was about to make some serious decisions at work, so she was delighted to meet an astrologer. We made an appointment there and then. What impressed me from the outset was her ability to make a decision and act on it straight away – there was no hesitation. She is an attractive, engaging woman with a quick sense of humour. She carries herself well, walks tall, and engages directly with the world. She is not shy, has a discerning intelligence, and her boardroom skills and diplomacy were apparent from the start. She is egalitarian and fair in her appraisals of both herself and her colleagues, and considers herself to be doing well. When I met her she had been divorced for some time.

During her initial consultation, the discussion centred on her career and possible movements within the company. She held a fairly high position in a corporate environment, and she soon had to make decisions the consequences of which could lead her into a sideways career path as opposed to a preferred upward path. She felt that there was a risk in taking one of the opportunities on the table, as it might lead to a premature dead end, while the other path, though apparently upwardly mobile, was more difficult to maintain, as it meant competing with more qualified people – and there was a definite gender bias towards men. I made several predictions regarding her career, and she later contacted me to relay that I had been correct with timing and content and to set a date for a further consultation. The second time she came to see me, her agenda was slightly different. This time she wanted to know about her personal life, her relationships and her prospects for having children.

## The Natal Chart as a Lens on Fertility

In assessing natal charts for fertility, there are a number of factors to take into account. Chief among these are: physical health and condition of eggs, hormonal or endocrine function, regularity of menstrual cycle and ovulation, availability of a sexual partner (or access to donor sperm), and the subtler consideration of possible psychological inhibitions that might obstruct conception.

In Amanda's chart (Figure 3.1) the first thing to note is an Aquarius Ascendant, which in fertility work is interpreted as 'highly strung' and 'finely-tuned'. Lord of the Chart is Saturn in the 12th house, in rulership and in his Joy, and squaring the Midheaven. Amanda's strength in life comes from not revealing her agendas all at once but keeping something back and using her finely-tuned Ascendant to work out the state of play of the world in which she moves.

When she came to see me in late November 2002, Amanda was forty-two years old and hoping to adopt a child through a reputable agency. She was looking for reassurance that this would be possible, and if the astrology indicated that it would not come to pass, she would not take the next step, which was assessment by the social services as a potential parent. This process is invasive, and would entail interviews with her bosses and her colleagues, something she would gratefully avoid if the probability for successful adoption was low. So she asked the question of me: 'will I successfully adopt a child?'

In talking with her about her history around children and pregnancy, she revealed an intriguing biography. Early in her life, she had met a man in another country on a holiday, had a romantic fling and came home unexpectedly pregnant. She had no way of knowing if this romance would develop into anything further, as the man in question was working and

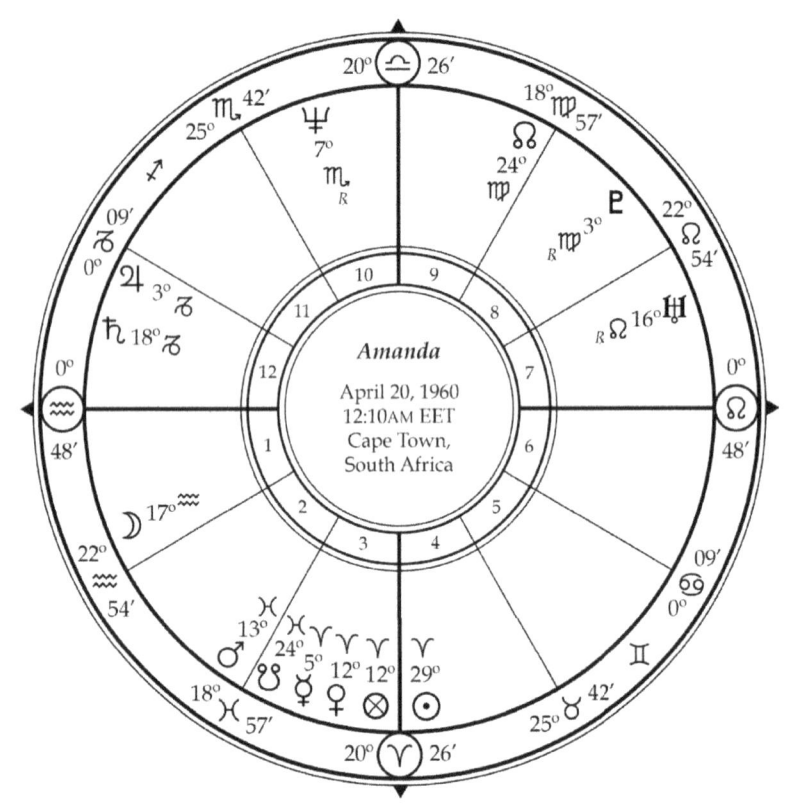

Figure 3.1: Amanda

living abroad, so in the absence of a future guarantee and while working hard to establish her own career, she decided to terminate the pregnancy. Some months later, he moved to her country to be with her, and they married. In time, she tried to fall pregnant again. She fell pregnant on two occasions but miscarried fairly early on each occasion. Due to pressure from her husband's family because of her failure to provide an heir, the marriage disintegrated, and he left to find work in another country. She remained, built a fabulous career, and tried off and on with donor sperm to get pregnant, as she deeply desired to be a mother. After many years of unsuccessful treatments, Amanda decided that adoption was now her last hope. And so, against this backdrop, we began our consultations.

## Dealing with Termination Guilt

The first time Amanda saw me, we spoke at length about her termination and that she had not told her husband about it. I gently introduced the possibility that her guilt surrounding the decision might have affected her subsequent attempts. She was able to consider this with an attitude of open and positive interest, and was relieved to finally be able to talk about it without fear of being judged for her actions. Pluto in the 8th house does not always imply terminations, but here it seemed apropos given her grand trine involving the Sun, Jupiter and Pluto – her ability to act impulsively, and to be able to destroy and simultaneously rebuild while maintaining her power in the world.

At this point, it is important to mention that in consultation a subtle shift of energy arising from either a statement from the astrologer 'hitting a nerve', or the client finally relaxing and being able to tell their story without inhibition, often signifies the arrival of the real matter at hand. Clients often come to ask ostensibly about one subject (career) and end up talking about another subject entirely (a chaotic relationship with their mother, for example). When this happens it is important to pay attention, for then the chart begins to 'sing', and the signatures come alive.[39] Talking about Amanda's termination was the way into her chart, a change of pace, an exchange. Amanda 'gave' me something, and in return the astrology came easily, without me struggling to manipulate the signatures to fit a particular narrative.

On reflection, Amanda was invoking the myth of Inanna/Ereshkigal. Like Inanna, she came to my room, shed her garments, revealed herself, and made herself vulnerable. Then, like Ereshkigal, she gave me her story of termination – of the pain, self-destruction and self-loathing. I am exaggerating the drama to demonstrate that some of your clients will go through the motions of the original myth: they lose something and have to give themselves up in order to be brought back into the light. It is a fulfilling experience as a therapist or astrologer to be conscious of the process that the client is going through, just as it is vital for us to hold their pain like the Kurgarra and Galatur, grieving with them. Ereshkigal and Inanna are one and the same; they are the sister sides of the planet Venus to astrologers, and when Venus is high in the sky she walks as Inanna. When she is dark and destructive with pain she is Ereshkigal, and it is the job of the astrologer to take the client to the light, but first to hear without judgement their painful past. In this way, the fertility myths are still very real in our practice, in addition to more typical chart symbolism.

Returning to her chart, Amanda's power as an Aries angular Sun comes from the 4th house. Her ambition to be a parent and so to build a family is apparent in the chart, and the wide square to Saturn in the 12th, ruler of the chart, suggests a certain aptitude in achieving her goals. Saturn, however, also squares her Venus (a little closer in orb) and her Part of Fortune, so her success seems to come only after a struggle and a certain amount of loss. A Venus in Aries can behave in a non-conformist way, being in detriment. Detriment, as described by Bernadette Brady, is when a planet is in exile – far away from home and in the company of foreigners, at odds with the current trends, different from others in the environment.[40] Amanda's rash and impulsive Venus will benefit from being expressed in a way that is different from the norm, or slightly at odds with society's expectations. This is something to remember for later. Her expectation of a normal relationship or marriage will have to be managed sensitively, and her natal Moon/Uranus opposition will also play a role in how successfully she can function in the mainstream.

The ruler of her Sun, Mars, is not strongly placed – in Pisces, in the 2nd house, and largely unaspected except for a wide sextile to Saturn in the 12th house. In the 2nd house of material wealth and self-esteem, Mars determines the motivation and ambition of her Sun in Aries. Her way of manifesting wealth or pursuing ambition (Mars also rules Part of Fortune) will be through visionary, trend-spotting projects, or the use of unorthodox methods, systems out of society's norm. So far, we have gone over the techniques you are probably familiar with. My next steps involve some you might not know yet.

When I prepare for a consultation, I like to start by examining the life of the native in general. I usually direct the Ascendant and the main luminary by triplicity, and then I will determine the Almuten of Pregnancy and direct that by triplicity as well. One of the most prominent writers about directing by triplicity is Dorotheus of Sidon, a first century Phoenician astrologer who wrote in Arabic. In the first chapter of his book *Carmen Astrologicum* he states:

> I tell you that everything which is decided or indicated is from the lords of the triplicities and as for everything of afflictions and distress

which reaches the people of the world and the totality of men, the lords of the triplicities decide it, in an eclipse of the Sun or the Moon in which they indicate the things that will happen and for how long it will be and of what kind it will be.[41]

The rest of the text is full of examples as to how he uses the three triplicity rulers of each planet (as well as the house cusp, Arabic part and even the hyleg, Ascendant, and Part of Fortune), to determine the flow of life or events linked to the signification of that particular chart point.

Directing by triplicity is a method of dividing the life of the native into three distinct chapters, and each chapter of life can indicate an improvement or a depreciation of health, wealth, relationship, etc. The length and time of each of these chapters of life, is determined by the length of life given by the astrologer to the native using the Alcocoden. So, for example, if the astrologer calculates that the life of the native is going to be seventy years, then one would divide the number of years by three and interpret the nature of those years by delineating the condition of the three triplicity rulers. Since Dorotheus was probably one of the earliest writers on triplicity rulership, the table below has come to be known as 'The Dorothean Triplicities'. Both Masha'allah and Guido Bonatti borrow this concept directly from Dorotheus, according to an article by Robert Zoller.[42]

Neither the *Carmen Astrologicum* nor Bonatti discuss directing an almuten by triplicity, but in light of the precedent set by Dorotheus to direct nearly every point in the chart by triplicity, I put forward a suggestion that one could (and indeed I do) direct the Almuten of Pregnancy in the same way. Doing this produces three distinct phases of fertility throughout one's life, regardless of whether one is male or female. That is, I direct this almuten in male charts as well.

Dorotheus favoured using the main luminary depending on whether or not the chart is nocturnal or diurnal. He emphasises the ability to express solar essence – even through the Moon in a nocturnal chart – as the greatest indicator of the flow of life. Bonatti, according to Zoller, favoured using the Ascendant as a means of ascertaining the health of the individual, as he equated good health with good circumstances. I use both, since I differentiate between a general upswing in financial or social circumstances and the state of someone's health; bad health no longer means an inevitably miserable life, and financial straits have never been an inhibitor of fertility.

So, using the Dorothean triplicities table below (Figure 3.2), we would say that the ruler of the first part of Amanda's life with regard to her health is the first of the air triplicities, since the Ascendant is ruled by Aquarius, which is Mercury; the second part of her life regarding her health is Saturn, and the last part of her life regarding health will be Jupiter. If it is a diurnal chart, the first triplicity ruler in the sequence would be used first, but since Amanda's chart is nocturnal, we use the second ruler first, then the first ruler, then the participating ruler.

| Triplicity | Day Rulers | | | Night Rulers | | |
|---|---|---|---|---|---|---|
| ♈ ♌ ♐ | ☉ | ♃ | ♄ | ♃ | ☉ | ♄ |
| ♉ ♍ ♑ | ♀ | ☽ | ♂ | ☽ | ♀ | ♂ |
| ♊ ♎ ♒ | ♄ | ☿ | ♃ | ☿ | ♃ | ♄ |

Figure 3.2: Dorothean Triplicities

Of course in earlier times the astrologer would have calculated the length of life first and, on that calculation, would have been able to be quite specific about when these rulership periods begin and end. I tend to assign each phase of life thirty years (for a total of ninety) as a general rule of thumb. Just to be clear, when we talk about directing the fertile life by triplicity, we are referring to the triplicities of the Almuten of Pregnancy, versus, for example the whole life which uses the triplicities of the Ascendant or main luminary.

Returning to Amanda's chart: she is forty-two years old, so we can assume she is in the second part of her life. Thus we would say that Saturn rules her health. Saturn looks pretty strong to me. It is in rulership, in his Joy, not retrograde, with the greater benefic Jupiter, and aspecting the MC. The triplicity rulers of her Moon (which we use because it is a nocturnal chart) are the same. So the triplicity ruler for her life in general in this phase is Saturn – again, really strong. Even if we took Ptolemy's preference for the Sun, we would find that her triplicity rulers are Jupiter, Sun, Saturn. Her Sun is angular, in exaltation, in the same house as her Part of Fortune, and square the Ascendant. So we might also say that she is looking strong in this phase, and while her health might suffer to some extent with the square of her Sun to the Ascendant, this is not likely to be a disaster, since the Sun is so strong. So, in general her health is good, and her life is upwardly mobile. All systems go.

## The Almuten of Pregnancy

The next step, when looking at fertility, is to see which planet has the most to say about the potential for pregnancy. Instead of playing a guessing game and making a prediction solely based on the ruler of the 5th house, there is a system that takes into account all the factors that work together in a chart to influence a viable pregnancy. In medieval astrology, calculating an almuten is a method that uses all the points and planets in a chart that might have a say in the outcome of a topic, in order to determine a winning planet, the almuten, which has the most say over that specific topic and can be used to make accurate predictions regarding it. Here we are concerned with conception, and in his *Book of Nativities*, Omar of Tiberias gives us the formula for calculating the Almuten of Pregnancy: the Ascendant and its ruler, the 5th house cusp and its ruler, the Moon and its ruler, the position of Jupiter, and so on.[43] All these factors are tabulated, and the degree points listed and then weighed according to a point system according to essential dignity: 5 points for rulership; 4 for exaltation; 3 for each triplicity ruler (each planet gets three points); 2 for term; and 1 point for face. When all the scores are added up, one planet will have the highest score, and that planet becomes the Almuten of Pregnancy. The calculations for Amanda's Almuten of Pregnancy look like the table on the following page (Figure 3.3).[44]

Saturn has the highest score, so Saturn is the almuten. As we know, Saturn is cadent, but joys in the 12th, is in rulership, and sitting with Jupiter the greater benefic in the sign of Capricorn. Jupiter is in fall in Capricorn and, according to Brady, the concept of fall can be understood as follows:

> the difference between detriment and fall is hard to judge in a natal chart. However, the planet in detriment is one that has not lost anything, but rather has problems achieving in the eyes of other people whereas *a planet in fall has the feel of the deposed conqueror, the one who has lost the crown, hence there may be an element of disgrace.*

## 32  Fertility Astrology

| POINT ON CHART | ☉ | ☿ | ☽ | ♀ | ♂ | ♃ | ♄ |
|---|---|---|---|---|---|---|---|
| ASC | | | | | | | |
| 8 deg Aq | | 3 | | 2+1 | | 3 | 5+3 |
| RULER OF ASC | | | | | | | |
| Saturn 18 deg Cap | | | 3 | 3+2 | 3+4 | 1 | 5 |
| MOON | | | | | | | |
| 17 deg Aq | | 3 | | | | 3+2 | 5+3 |
| RULER OF MOON | | | | | | | |
| Saturn 18 deg Cap | | | 3 | 3+2 | 3+4+1 | | 5 |
| 5TH CUSP | | | | | | | |
| 25 deg Tau | | | 3+4 | 5+3 | 3 | | 1+2 |
| RULER OF 5TH | | | | | | | |
| Venus 12 deg Aries | 4+3+1 | 2 | | | 5 | 3 | 3 |
| POSITION JUP | | | | | | | |
| 3 deg Capricorn | | 2 | 3 | 3 | 4+3 | 1 | 5+3 |
| PLANETS IN 5TH | | | | | | | |
| None | | | | | | | |
| TOTALS | 8 | 10 | 16 | 24 | 30 | 13 | 40 |

Figure 3.3: Calculating Amanda's Almuten of Pregnancy

The condition of being in fall was considered a greater depletion than detriment.[45]

It didn't surprise me that Amanda was pregnant before, given that Jupiter in fall is conjunct the Almuten of Pregnancy; and our understanding of her sense of guilt at having terminated can now be deepened: she realises that she had chosen to lose something she once held in the palm of her hand, and is now slightly edgy about whether or not she deserves another chance. Amanda's Saturn is also in the terms of Venus. *The Liber Hermetis*, attributed to Hermes Trismegistus, interprets this as follows:

> The Mother 'digs the child from her womb'. Mother dies before the father and the person may see the death of their daughter and or wife. They will become head of the family – lord of their father's house – and acquire much then lose it later. They will be a difficult person to deal with and may well raise a family containing their own children as well as those of others.[46]

So whatever else Saturn brings to the table in terms of pregnancy, being the Almuten it will inevitably involve loss, termination, or 'blended' families. Parenthood is emphasised as something that is hard come by, or, not given easily in the chart.

Now, by directing the Almuten according to triplicity, we see that the first part of Amanda's fertile life is ruled by the Moon, the second by Venus and the last by Mars in an earth sign. The Moon is not particularly stable; it is strong enough in the 1st house, but opposed by an outer planet, and by tradition not at all happy when ruled by Saturn. However, in Amanda's case, where Saturn is the Almuten of Pregnancy, this Moon fairs well despite the instability. The opposition to Uranus might indicate early, sudden, unpredictable pregnancy, but, seeing as Uranus had yet to be discovered in medieval times, there is no evidence in any of the early traditional texts to support this interpretation. Physically, her menstrual cycle could have been erratic given the opposition to Uranus, but she assured me that her cycle was regular and normal. Emotionally, she agreed that she was a bit up and down in those earlier years, and that she did suffer some uncertainty regarding her ability to mother a child as a single parent, hence the termination.

The second part of her fertile life is ruled by Venus in detriment, but Venus is strengthened by being very close to the IC, conjunct the Part of Fortune, and in proximity to the very powerful angular Sun. So, given Venus' detriment, it would be fairly safe to assume that success in fertility would come from unusual events and alternative treatments and definitely not with the sanction of society, and more than likely in the second part of her life.

The third part of her fertile life is largely irrelevant. For Amanda, as for most women, it is extremely uncommon to have babies at the age of sixty plus, so considering that by this time most women are well into menopause, I hardly ever need to pay attention to directing the third part of life or the Almuten of Pregnancy to determine the possible success of fertility treatment.

In Amanda's chart her triplicity ruler for the second part of her life is Saturn, coincidentally also the Almuten of Pregnancy, which means that it is in the second part of her life that she will be most successful. As stated previously, Saturn is well placed and has high status given that he is the Almuten of Pregnancy. When I note that the planet that is the significator of the Almuten of Pregnancy is the ruler of the second part of her life, and that the second triplicity ruler of that Almuten is also strongly placed (Venus conjunct the 4th house, Part of Fortune and Sun, in aspect to Saturn, the Almuten of Pregnancy), understandably I get quite excited.

## A Thorough Delineation of the Astrology in Amanda's Chart

### Her Moon

Her 1st house Moon gives her a good public profile, emotional stability and a receptive quality to both her appearance and her physical body. Her Moon is in opposition to Uranus, in the 7th house, and her ability to tune into her entire 7th house – business partners and husbands – is something that she can build on. Emotionally speaking, she tells me that in her personal life, she suffers from 'love it/hate it' syndrome. She finds it hard to commit to something unless she has an out-clause, and she finds personal relationships hard work since she requires a higher than average degree of independence. This marker indicates someone who is emotionally detached, unattainable, and unpredictable, who has a fierce need for independence. Because the need for freedom is so paramount, single life is often the only real option. Commitment is difficult, and the need for a relationship is virtually non-existent, which both intrigues and confuses people, who assume that someone who doesn't need a partner is somehow flawed. Fertility is going to be an issue for anyone who lives with this kind of emotional tension and constant drive to assert independence.

Now let's consider the biological parameter. With Amanda's Moon in the 1st house, and in the sign of the Ascendant, which is in her Sun's detriment, it would be prudent to explore her menstrual cycle, which we might expect to be irregular, given the ticklish opposition to Uranus. If an astrologer suggests that a woman with such a Moon might have irregular periods, while the client insists that her cycle is perfectly punctual every twenty-eight days, then we will likely find that although she might bleed every twenty-eight days, her ovulation cycle, that is the releasing of her eggs each month, might be irregular. So thinking that ovulation happens on the fourteenth day and having sexual intercourse then may not achieve success. Women with Moon in Aquarius, or in the 1st house ruled by

Aquarius, need to be aware that they might need to be scanned each month to see exactly when the egg matures and is released. It could be that one month they ovulate on day eight and on the next, day nineteen. Any remedy taken then is going to seem haphazard and ineffectual.

Amanda reported a regular cycle, but she was not sure when she ovulated, so treatments such as artificial insemination and other natural home methods are tricky, without scanning each and every month. Ridder-Patrick supports this statement, observing:

> Psychologically this aspect is associated with the sense of a lack of stability and security, where emotional upheaval is felt to be possible at any moment and nurturing is inconsistent and unreliable. There is often intense emotional excitability, which is greatest in the fire signs. This is combined with sensitivity, a highly-strung nature and nervous tension. There can be erratic and overwhelming emotional outbursts. The resulting high-tension, emotional 'electricity' needs to be grounded, and the person soothed and centred by periods of quiet and relaxation in which the charged feelings can be processed and assimiliated. Otherwise it is possible that a breakdown in health might occur due to the prolonged over-stimulation of the nervous system. There may be a link with autism and Asperger's syndrome, especially if the Moon is in Aquarius.[47]

Further, she states, 'There can be menstrual irregularities, pain at ovulation and dysmenorrhea. It can lead to colic in any fluid-excreting or fluid-containing organ [...] as well as disturbances in blood pressure'.[48] Although Ridder-Patrick suggests here someone who is outwardly emotionally volatile, it must be noted that quite often Moon/Uranus aspects include emotional instability that is not obvious to others because of the ability that some Moon/Uranus people have to effectively disassociate themselves from emotions that threaten to overwhelm them. So while they may *present* as calm and in control, they are in fact internally juggling strong emotional tides. It is up to the fertility astrologer to determine how much of the aspect may be internalised, and therefore manifested in terms of lifestyle or personality rather than in physical reality as expressed through the body.

A biographical note on Amanda's mother: she had two children, both daughters. At the time of the consultation, Amanda's mother was considered old, in her late eighties, and it was clear she had conceived her children late in life, compared to her peer group.

Finally, Saturn ruling Amanda's Moon might suggest that the outer lining of the egg is also too hard for the sperm to penetrate, in which case IVF with ICSI is the only remedial treatment indicated.

**Her Sun**
Her Sun, in its exaltation in Aries and angular in the 4th, square the Ascendant, is well placed for a high degree of visibility in the world and a strong potential for success. It is in the same sign as the Part of Fortune, conjunct Venus. This is clearly an ambitious, no nonsense person, whose material success is self-motivated, and cardinal. Her issues in life will concern home and hearth, name and genealogy; making a secure base for herself to be able to express her vital, solar essence from a platform of confidence in her heritage, and to create home and family for herself, in which she can express her deep desire to care and nurture others.

The 4th house is the traditional house of the father, not the mother, and although there are some who would disagree and could present many valid reasons for the 10th being the house of father, I practise medieval and traditional astrology, and I stick to that interpretive tradition here. Amanda's issues can then be refined to include those related to the father in the home, his place in it, what impact it has on her, and, finally, her decisions related to parenting. Her Sun is in a wide square to Saturn in the 12th, and this would further suggest issues with a parent, and possibly the father since the square is coming off the 4th and 12th houses. One could go into more detail and make suggestions such as, this parent, who seemingly has a huge impact on her, is also fairly invisible in the 12th house, suggesting that they are possibly in an institution (such as prison), missing, or for whatever reason, not available to her. This parent does not seem overly malefic, since Saturn is in rulership, and in its Joy, not retrograde; however, he is out of sect. One could say that this parent is absent for long periods of time, but leaves behind a strong moral or guiding principle; or that the outcome of such emotional distance causes the native to rely on her own moral compass and create her own guiding principles regarding the establishment of a home and solid foundation.

Her Ascendant is in her Sun's detriment, so there is a fair degree of conflict between her environment and her Sun's ability to be itself.

There are a number of ways this could play out. Amanda could choose environments where she does not fit in, and therefore by default does not conform to her father's way of life. Another possibility is that, by virtue of not having him in her life, she could choose environments where she is considered the norm, only because the rules are different. Or, due to her Sun's ambition to become a mother, she could put herself outside of the norm in her environment or Ascendant. One way or another, she will find herself outside the norm.

**Her Venus**

I have mentioned detriment now several times and it would seem that Amanda's chart is teeming with planets in fall, detriment or peregrine: Mars, Venus, Jupiter are all in *difficult* placements, and her Ascendant is in her Sun's detriment. Her functioning in the world requires her to be always outside of the tribe, different from her peer group, and in relationships that do not conform to any normal 'rules', etc. In medieval times, this would have meant a life of hardship, exile, and being excluded from the clan, consequently being deprived of resources necessary for social and physical nurturing and expression. In short, she would have been excommunicated because of her desire for personal liberation and freedom. She would have been found wanting as marriage material. Her natal Venus in Aries is far too passionate and impulsive. She would not have been considered chaste, according to the draconian rules of the past, and she might have lost her life because of it.

However, in 2002 things were a little different. She had developed a reputation for her entrepreneurial skills, and she enjoyed a corporate working life that involved travel, a huge portfolio of responsibility, and a network of peers that valued the different perspective she brought to the table. In a world where differentiation equals trendsetting, businesses based in marketing or packaging or presentation benefit from employing people like Amanda. She knew what it was to have a different value system, she understood what it was like to be different, and she turned this medieval affliction – detriment – into a veritable source of income for herself. Her need to marry (to secure material security and status) decreased as she found herself the CEO of an international organization; she had status in a male-dominated world and material success to support her independent lifestyle. This is a perfect manifestation of her Venus conjunct the Part of Fortune in the 4th – creating home and hearth for herself outside of society's norms or expectations, successfully and with the spirit of adventure.

The square from Venus to Saturn is alarming at first, until one realises that Saturn is not in such bad shape and is the Almuten of Pregnancy. This aspect is one of unrequited love, elusive intimacy, absent lovers, long distance relationships and great psychological distance between intimate partners. Amanda could not function if her life was bound up with that of an intimate partner; it would threaten her Moon, it would make her Ascendant even more highly strung and her independent spirit would be stifled in a soul-binding partnership. So, this square is perfect in the space it creates for her to be not in need of a 'soulmate' or otherwise entwined relationship. She finds partners who are equally desirous of independent relationships, and she finds that the compromise is just that one does not always feel deeply connected all the time to one's partner, although she feels sometimes melancholic that the Hallmark card version of romance is nearly always unavailable to her as a life experience.

When Amanda came to see me the second time, we had already explored these interpretations in detail and her biography had provided enough substantial evidence to support all of the above.

**The Power of Mercury**

With all fertility clients, and indeed especially with every young woman I see, I investigate the condition of Mercury carefully in order to establish the condition of her fallopian tubes. I don't mean to suggest that Mercury rules the fallopian tubes due to the fact that the tubes are a 'way travelled' by the egg, or that the tubes 'connect' the ovaries with the uterus – this would be, for my purposes, an over-simplistic rulership system. Writers in this area will, of course, differ in their interpretive emphases according to their different purposes.

Eileen Nauman, for example – whose book on holistic medical astrology incorporates asteroids, transneptunian planets and midpoints, Bach flower remedies and more – mentions the fallopian tubes specifically only once:

> Mercury rules Gemini; consequently, with a Sun-Mercury conjunction there can be various disorders related to the Gemini-directed tubes of the body, such as the eustachian tubes of the ears, the bronchial

tubes of the lungs, the ureters leading from the kidneys to the bladder, the urethra leading from the bladder to the outer openings, the fallopian tubes carrying eggs from the ovaries to the uterus and the cerebrospinal system.[49]

Nauman uses Mercury as the ruler of a 'way travelled', rather than the more alchemical approach that I favour. While undergoing my own fertility treatment, it occurred to me that since fertilisation of the egg and the sperm happens in the fallopian tube, it is the place or location of the 'cosmic marriage' of the solar and lunar principle (sperm and egg). So Mercury facilitates, on an alchemical principle, the coming together of sperm and egg to form the embryo, which then travels to the uterus; the uterus either accepts or rejects the embryo, and conception happens. This realisation led me to consider that the condition and dignity of Mercury in every chart is significant, that every placement has a comment to make on the essential condition of the fallopian tubes. In addition, if one's thinking (Mercury) is in detriment – out of the mainstream, contra to society's norm – then the choice of sexual partner and orientation towards childbearing will be part of that expression. There are two placements for Mercury to be in detriment (in Pisces and in Sagittarius), and consequently, approximately 16 percent of all charts have this placement.

Mercury combust the Sun is frequently present with ectopic pregnancies, where the embryo embeds itself in the fallopian tube and not in the uterus – a dangerous and life-threatening condition, which usually results in an emergency operation to remove the offending tube. A Mesopotamian interpretation of this combust placement could be that the conception takes place in 'the other place' – which is of course the only other place it could embed itself. Mercury with Neptune has presented with damage to the fallopian tubes due to untreated STIs, for example Chlamydia, which is silent and can appear after one episode of sexual activity. Mercury with Uranus most frequently indicates a laparoscopy (small incision to the abdomen to investigate or operate on the tube), and also suggests the potential for IVF treatment – fertilization through technology and surgery.

There is a distinct interpretation for each and every placement of Mercury in a chart, and a fertility astrologer should carefully investigate this as a source of helpful information that cannot be seen without medical intervention. For women who are only starting to have families in their forties, saving time in fertility treatment is a major part of the battle.

So, in Amanda's chart, her Mercury is conjunct Venus, well placed, angular, conjunct the Part of Fortune, and free of combustion. There is nothing irregular about her fallopian tubes and indeed her previous naturally conceived pregnancy supports this. I have no further need to investigate here.

**Orienting Amanda More Effectively Towards Motherhood**

The main thrust of the remedial part of the consultation was aimed at helping Amanda overcome the trauma of her previous termination and bringing in new energy to her 5th house, which is ruled by a very fixed sign, Taurus. I wanted Amanda to experiment with creativity, and I wanted her to bring into her 5th house some moist and warm 'humours' in the form of watercolour, oil painting or ceramics. My suggestion was that she should get in touch with her creative muscles, start to flex them, and choose a medium that involved a blank canvas, so that form and shape had to come from deep within her subconscious, as she worked with moist materials, all of Venus' palette of colour. She took up oil painting and returned the next month, quite pleased with her efforts and proud of her work.

The role of ritual should not be underestimated in the 'treatment'. Making small changes in daily routine, consciously taking time and effort to shift something in the material world, can help facilitate the shift in the spiritual world. Even simple measures can produce results. For example, you could suggest to your clients the following remedy: every time you use or see water – in the bath or sink, or in a pond or stream – simply connect with the thought that water is a life-giving, fertile gift. While you swirl your hands in the water, imagine that you are touching the fertile creative matrix that gives life to all living things. Suggestions such as this are part of what I referred to in the second chapter – it is an opportunity to create meaning and intent for the client. It will help focus the client on what they would like to achieve, and it also gives them a feeling of being in control or that they have something concrete to do. In the field of infertility, this is essential.

At the next consultation, where I was to give Amanda a conclusive answer to the question of whether or not she would adopt a child, I confronted my biggest challenge to date as a practising astrologer. A simple horary chart or a simple transit were not enough to lead me to a conclusion. Remember that I was making a prediction for a woman who was forty-two years old, approaching menopause, had no sexual partner in her life, had tried to conceive for eight previous years without success, and was desperate to avoid social embarrassment at work, and simultaneously desperate to mother a child.

## A Surprise Gift from Jupiter…

In the unpacking of her chart, an upcoming transit of Jupiter to her natal Uranus in her 7th house caused me to pause and to think about what benefic gift or blessing could be coming to her (Jupiter opposes her Moon by transit) and her ex-husband (Uranus in the 7th). In looking at her chart, I dismissed all other interpretations for Jupiter, simply because I was looking for a baby, not a book, not overseas travel or higher learning. So I took this idea (that something Jupiterian was coming to both her ex and herself) a little further, and asked her where her ex-husband was at that moment. She said he lived in another country, that they spoke a couple of times a year, but that she had little or no contact with him on a regular basis.

Bearing in mind that Saturn, Almuten of Pregnancy, was the triplicity ruler on two counts for this period in her life and, moreover, was transiting through her 5th house at the time, I ventured a prediction that she would not adopt, but that she would likely get pregnant at the same time as her ex-husband, and if she was really lucky, she would get pregnant with his baby. The reason for the breakup of their marriage was that she could not achieve pregnancy and a live birth with him, and the idea of a sexual relationship with him again was not repulsive to her in the least; in fact she welcomed the idea, it seemed to have a correctness about it. She said she would prefer his child to donor sperm, but that she had also not had luck with his sperm in the past.

Her profected ruler for her forty-second year was the Sun, which natally is angular, conjunct Venus and Mercury, and aspecting Saturn, the Almuten of Pregnancy, so it isn't surprising that this is the year she decided to take charge of her desire for a child and that there is strong indication of success. There is also strong indication that she will achieve success through her 7th house (ex-husband) and redefine her relationship with him. In the solar return for her forty-second year, the chart ruler was Jupiter in Cancer (its exaltation) conjunct the Moon (wide) and applying to the 5th house. Quite a fertile signature.

## Checking Fixed Stars

As a last step in my delineation, I always check fixed stars, as the starlore associated with certain stars provides my consultations with valuable prognostic details. Using the Starlight software program, I checked to see which fixed stars, if any, were in parans to this transiting Jupiter, both for the natal location and for the location of her ex-husband.[50] For transiting Jupiter I found, in the mundane parans for the location of the conception:

> Jupiter – Type of Action which is Favoured by this Period of Time
>
> *On Nadir when Alderamin is Culminating orb 00 mins 05 secs –*
> Act with great dignity and take the moral high ground
> *Culminating when Alderamin is on Nadir orb 00 mins 15 secs –*
> Act with great dignity and take the moral high ground
> *Rising when Thuban is Rising orb 00 mins 58 secs –*
> Release all information, have no secrets
> *On Nadir when Capella is Rising orb 01 mins 26 secs –*
> Fast action, bold insights

Capella is a star in the constellation of the crook of the great Hunter, Orion, and this is Brady's interpretation of the significance of that star:

> The need for independence: Capella in most charts lends a nurturing but free-spirited flavour. The star is linked to Artemis the Greek goddess of the hunt as her Roman counterpart Diana. It is the concept of the fertile goddess but she is of the horse and therefore embodies action and movement. With Capella in paran with one of your planets you will have issues to do with freedom and independence in a non-aggressive way. There will be a need for freedom.[51]

It is worth remembering that Amanda was seeking to have a child, while still 'riding her horse' in a male dominated world, and while maintaining her independence at the same time.

Then, I always make sure to look to the condition and parans of Mercury in fertility charts because, as I have mentioned before, Mercury-Hermes has to facilitate the cosmic marriage. Mercury is also the doctor performing the treatment, as well as, of course, the astrologer. The parans to Mercury on that day were striking in their accuracy:

> *Rising when CASTOR is Setting* [...]
>> To present a good or clever plan
>
> *Setting when SIRIUS is Rising* [...]
>> A publication, or the words of a person, have far-reaching repercussions
>
> *Rising when POLLUX is Setting* [...]
>> An opinion voiced which goes against the tide of public thinking

As a theme for the day at the location of her conception, the Sun had the following stars in parans:

> *Rising when SPICA is Culminating* [...]
>> A bright idea, a new solution
>
> *On Nadir when SIRIUS is Culminating* [...]
>> The potential for great and immortal events to unfold
>
> *Rising when FACIES is Rising* [...]
>> The piercing stare of an aggressor or a critic

It would be superfluous to unpack these simple phrases of interpretation from Starlight. It is interesting, however, to consider the myth of the constellation Orion and the star Sirius in a fertility context. In *Brady's Book of Fixed Stars*, she writes about the story:

> The goddess Isis was the wife of Osiris (constellation Orion), the great god who was the first to be swallowed by precession into the whirlpool. In mythology he is killed and his body dismembered. Isis in mourning travelled through the land and found all the pieces of his body and, binding them together, she brought him back to life long enough to impregnate her with their son Horus (Aldebaran in the constellation of Taurus), who later became heir to the throne.[52]

There are some other translations of this myth that are more specific in their description of Isis actually sewing Osiris's genitalia back together (in some myths, Isis fashions a prosthetic phallus) for the purpose of conceiving. This aspect of the myth easily lends itself to the suggestion of Sirius as a potential significator for IVF and other fertility treatments. The fact that Sirius becomes the heliacal rising star at the same time that the Nile floods the valley with fertile, life-giving water is yet another reason to attribute fertile signatures when this star is in parans or on the angles in a chart.

Finally, I look to the parans of the Moon for good measure, since it is the Moon who, according to Ptolemy, deposits the soul on earth on the preventional or conjunctional lunation, the lunation prior to birth. Her Moon only made one paran, with the star Ankaa on the Nadir, which shows 'Concern with the wellbeing of families'. Brady interprets this significance as follows:

> Transcending, transforming. Not a great deal of work has been done with this star but it does seem to carry a sense of transformation or transcending. So look at the planet that this star is linked to and recognise that in that area of your life you will encounter transformations that can lead to a true transcending experience. It is in this part of your life that you can truly change or alter things around you, not through force and action, but via insights that transcend.[53]

Amanda was now in a position to totally transform her usually unstable Moon into the receptive and nurturing maternal expression which had always eluded her. The combination of all of these parans working together brings certain conditions into being. It is important to remember that it is not just one star in one paran that operates as a trigger. Stars rise and set at different locations (latitude) as opposed to time (longitude), and it is the stars which dictate the kind of energy that 'walks with the mortals' each day at each location. So there are places of gladness and of sadness, places of peace and of turmoil, places of industry, and, even places where babies are made, all over the world at different times. The trick in fertility astrology is getting your client to the place where babies are!

Given all this, so as to narrow down the best possible timing for Amanda to conceive, I chose the exact transit of Jupiter to her natal

Uranus, adjusted for her probable menstrual cycle, and said that 8 January 2003 looked like a good date for conception.

**Other support from the gods**
Now other transits and solar arcs revealed their support for Jupiter's nod. Transiting Jupiter stayed at 16 degrees of Leo for the first ten days of January, after reaching exactness on 31 December 2002 at 16 degrees 56 mins Rx. To stay within a degree or two of her natal Uranus for the rest of the month is an acceptably long conjunction of an outer planet. Transiting Venus was sextile her Moon/Jupiter midpoint on 3 January 2003, and conjunct the 11th house cusp at the same time. Significantly, the 11th house is her 7th house partner's 5th house by derived house system. In fact there was a Venus/Mars conjunction in the sky hovering on her 11th house cusp for that week. In addition on 15 January 2003, Saturn, her Almuten of Pregnancy, conjoined her Sun/Uranus midpoint in her 5th house.

The most notable and glaring indicator of them all has to be a solar arc direction for 18 January 2003 (day nineteen of her cycle), where solar arc Jupiter conjoined her Venus/Uranus midpoint in her 5th house. This was co-incidentally the day on which she would start producing pregnancy hormones, if the conception occurred, and if she had taken a blood sample on that day, there would have been a result.

The next day – 19 January 2003 – transiting Jupiter seemed to underline the Venus/Uranus midpoint with a sextile. I use midpoint theory and interpretations from Reinhold Ebertin's classic text *Combination of Stellar Influences* (*COSI*), and I have found that his interpretations yield strong results for my work.[54] *COSI* describes Jupiter conjunct Venus/Uranus midpoint as: 'The love of art, a sense of rhythm, inspired artistic receptivity', and 'A sudden and passing happiness in love, artistic success, birth'.[56] *COSI* describes the probable manifestations of such an aspect:

+ the tendency to be particular and fastidious in the choice of a partner or lover, passing love-bonds, romantic love inclinations, popularity, - Births.
- A love adventure, nervous troubles, unfaithfulness, - Births.

## Back to Earth…

Amanda listened patiently to my prediction and my astrological support before venturing the obvious: the ex-husband lived in another country, could have a girlfriend, was not planning to come to visit her, and she had no invitation to go to see him. They had tried to get pregnant before, and there was no reason to suppose that this time would be successful, especially since she was much older and possibly not ovulating as regularly as she had done in her youth.

I have to confess that there was a moment, during my investigation of her chart, where I felt that the story of her possible pregnancy 'came' to me. I definitely 'saw' the potential in the chart; my confidence in delivering the information to my client was supported by the astrology, but I had taken an intuitive leap to get there. Notwithstanding the seemingly obvious obstacles to this fantasy prediction of mine, I stood my astrological ground and said that I would see her again in a month, when I would have another look at the charts to see if I could find further direction.

On 10 December 2002, Amanda's ex-husband contacted her. He had heard that her sister had moved permanently to another country, and he was writing to say that this news had set him thinking of her and how lonely she might be, and would she like to come and visit him on the weekend of 8 January 2003. Now, even if she went to visit him and becoming pregnant turned out to be a self-fulfilling prophecy, then that in itself is miracle enough. But when she accepted his invitation, she didn't know whether or not he had a girlfriend, and she did know how hard it would be to reignite a relationship with an ex. It is in fact, much easier to sleep with a stranger than to renegotiate your way into an ex's bed, just for the sake of it, let alone for the purpose of getting pregnant. But she went, and at the retiring end of the evening (as she told me later) she just 'knew' she was going to succeed, since apparently the guest room bed had not been made up, and she had noticed that his body language was receptive to rekindling intimacy.

### The Results
She called me some time after she returned and said that they had spent a gorgeous weekend together (mostly in bed) and that she was five days

late in her menstrual cycle. That afternoon she saw a doctor, and the next day she confirmed she was pregnant!

A period of detailed research followed in the months to come, and by the time Amanda's son was born (23 September 2003), I had predicted seven more pregnancies almost to the day. It was a steep and intense learning curve, and it formed the basis of the kind of astrology I principally practise today.

Amanda told the father of her child about her condition when she was six months pregnant, he attended the birth and is a devoted and caring parent. He moved back to the city where she lives, and they shared a unique and innovative relationship for two or three years, so that Amanda could receive his help with their son, and they could both establish a bond with him – and each other.

**A Biographical Note on Amanda's Father**
Amanda's mother had an affair during her marriage, and Amanda was the result of that affair. Her mother had chosen not to tell the biological father, nor to disturb her marriage in any way, and eventually had another child, this time by her husband. Some years later, when Amanda's real father became ill, her mother finally told Amanda, who then went to see her biological father shortly before he passed away.

The astrology in Amanda's case finds another layer of richness in the postscript that Amanda nearly repeated this family narrative in her own life: she was initially reluctant to tell her ex-husband about the baby. It is also astrologically remarkable that Saturn in rulership in the 12th aptly describes a father who, though having power in the world, remains hidden, and this anomalous relationship somehow has a bearing on her need to rebuild family. In her own story, she does tell the father of her child, thereby finally healing the hidden, yet unresolved, wound of her own parentage – a 4th house Sun in Aries square Saturn. Amanda and her ex-husband are now in separate relationships, but they remain excellent friends and parents. Their son continues to bring them all great joy and happiness. A truly magnificent Sun/Venus/Part of Fortune conjunction on the IC.

## Conclusion

As a beginner it is tempting to leap upon the signatures that worked in a chart and want to repeat them with all future charts in the expectation that they should work in the same way. After all, Amanda fell pregnant on a transit of Jupiter to a 7th house planet, so why not interpret that all transits of Jupiter to planets in the 7th or cusp are also going to be fertile? In the next chapter we see that not all transits are equal; closer inspection reveals a much more unique pattern present in two very similar natal charts, both experiencing a transit of Jupiter to the 1st/7th axis and transiting planets in the 7th house.

## Notes

39. Gunzburg, Darrelyn. 'How Do Astrologers Read Charts?' *Astrologies: Plurality and Diversity*.
40. Brady, Bernadette. *Astro Logos – Medieval Astrology Certificate Study Guide*.
41. Dorotheus of Sidon, *Carmen Astrologicum*.
42. http://www.new-library.com/zoller/features/rz-article-arabic.shtml
43. Omar of Tiberias, *Three Books on Nativities*, p.89.
44. See Appendix Almuten Worksheet for a blank version.
45. Brady, *Medieval Astrology Study Guide*, p.17.
46. Hermes Trismegistus, *Liber Hermetis*, trans. Robert Zoller, p.68.
47. Ridder-Patrick, Jane. *A Handbook of Medical Astrology*, 2nd ed., p.76.
48. Ibid.
49. Eileen Nauman, *Medical Astrology*, third ed., p.36.
50. Brady, Bernadette. Barneswood Ltd, *Starlight: Returning the Stars to Astrology*, Version 1.0 (2002).
51. Ibid.
52. Brady, Bernadette. *Brady's Book of Fixed Stars*, pp.84–85.
53. *Starlight*.
54. Ebertin, Reinhold. *The Combination of Stellar Influences*. Hereafter *COSI*.
55. Ibid.

# 4

# Case Study – Nancy and Lisa
# Predictability and all its Complexity

Most critics of astrology like to point out that the same things don't happen to people born at the same time in the same place, and that the same events don't happen to everyone at the same location. And they are right. Life is not that simplistically predictable, and astrology cannot make it so – not because astrology doesn't work, but because its efficacy is drawn from a more complex understanding of 'predictability' than popularly supposed, and degrees of accuracy at this level of prediction depend on the calibre of the astrologer's skill and knowledge. All the same, this ever-hovering criticism does produce an occasional flutter of nervousness in even the most accomplished astrologer, and if we have the opportunity to provide a clear and unequivocal chart comparison in demonstration of just how it does work, we naturally snap it up. I offer such a clarifying comparison here.

## A Gift of Two Charts

In the course of my research, I looked for similar charts with similar transits in women undergoing IVF treatment on the same day at the same location. Amazingly, I have two charts, belonging to two different women, that fulfil these criteria, and what makes this data invaluable is that the same doctor performed the procedure minutes apart for both of these women, thus eliminating another subset of variables.

Nancy (Figure 4.1) and Lisa (Figure 4.2) made appointments with a fertility specialist at the same clinic in the same month. Nancy already had two children from a previous marriage, and now needed treatment to try for another with her second husband. Lisa had had three treatments in her attempt for a much-wanted first child with her husband.

50  Fertility Astrology

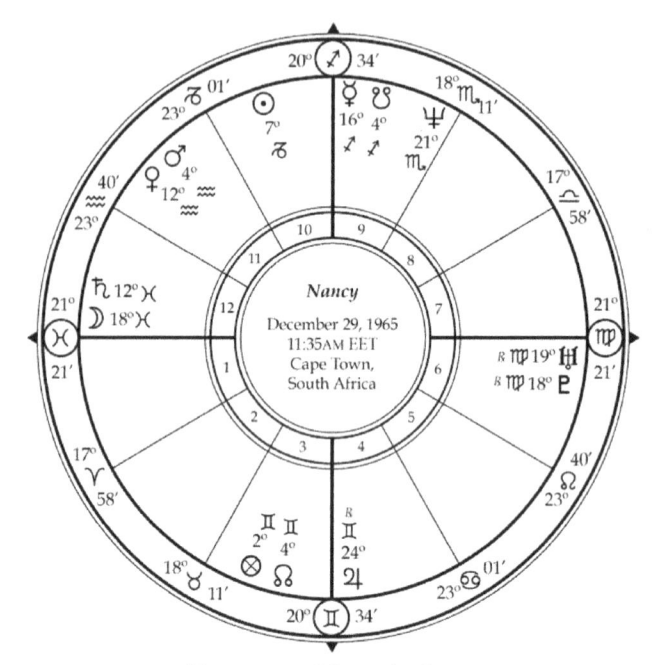

Figure 4.1: Nancy's chart

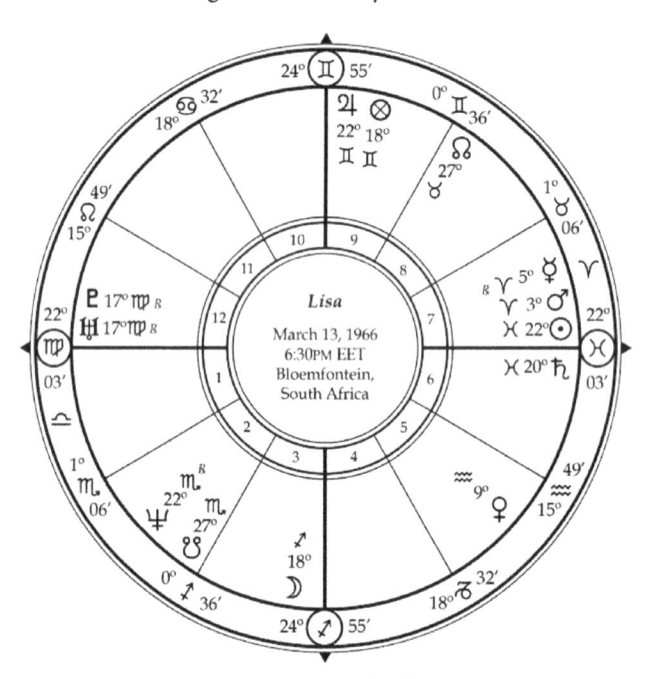

Figure 4.2: Lisa's chart

The similarities between these charts are breathtaking. Because these women were born only seventy-odd days apart, the outer planets are still making the same aspects to one another. The three points of the T-square between Jupiter, Saturn and Uranus/Pluto are generational, and therefore valid for a number of people born during those months at that location. In both charts, this T-square is angular, meaning that impacts or shifts in the collective will manifest on a quite physical level in the biographies of these women.

My interpretation of modern outer planets has shifted since I started using medieval astrological techniques. Outer planets are not personal planets, and they are malefic, in that they don't care at all for the person whose life they affect. They bring mayhem and destruction to whole generations of people in order to shift the collective and to radically change social patterns in large groups, countries, or minority groups. So, wicked though this Grand Cross looks in both charts (the Moon forms the fourth point in Lisa's chart and Mercury forms the fourth point in Nancy's chart), the Cross is not so much personally focused, as indicating more generally that Nancy and Lisa will involved in larger-frame activities that are indicated by the angularity and aspect pattern of these three outer planets.

The Saturn/Uranus opposition of the '60s in South Africa, where these two women were born, was a time of radical challenge to authority or patriarchy – in the rebellion against apartheid, in the finding of the 'self', and in the struggle for individual civic and human rights of black minority groups. In terms of human reproduction, several long-entrenched laws were challenged both in South Africa and worldwide: in 1970 Norma Corvey (aka Jane Roe) took on the American courts in challenge for the right of women to abortion on demand; Edwards and Steptoe (collaborating from 1968–78) published breakthroughs in fertility treatment techniques, as did Yanagamichi (1964) in Japan; and the contraceptive pill was in circulation.[56]

These two women were not excluded from the Saturn/Uranus narrative of the time. Nancy had been divorced (her natal Saturn/Uranus opposition falls in the 1st/7th houses), while Lisa preferred to live remotely on a farm cut off from neighbours. Both of them thus demonstrated their need to express a profound desire for personal and physical freedom and to create a sense of space in which to experience this. That they both signed up for fertility treatment is a further manifestation of the need to have a personal, physical experience of the reproductive issues of the time in which they were born.

In Lisa's chart, her Pisces Sun forms part of her Grand Cross, as does her Moon; this makes for a more challenging life, since both luminaries are involved on the angles. Nancy has an easier time, since her largely unaspected, accidentally dignified, 10th house Sun is not involved in the Grand Cross, so whatever issues her Pisces Moon has in relation to the Grand Cross might not affect her whole life, just her inner lunar private space. Remarkably, the angles in both charts are within a degree of one another, making any transiting aspect to these points open to a similar predictive interpretation. So, what makes these charts and their outcomes so different? Let us begin by examining their triplicity rulerships.

**Nancy**
In Nancy's chart, her Ascendant is in Pisces, so the triplicity rulerships for her sense of vitality (and in particular her health) and wellbeing are Venus, Mars, Moon (diurnal chart) according to the table of Dorothean triplicities. With reference to health, in the first phase of her life, Nancy enjoys good health, as indicated by a conjunction of Mars and Venus in the 11th house of good fortune, and the lack of aspects to malefics. Mars, the ruler of the second phase of her life, is in the fortunate 11th house, conjunct his consort Venus – and trine the Part of Fortune no less – so her health in the second part of her life looks good.

The triplicity rulers of the Sun – in the earth sign of Capricorn – are then, in sequence, Venus, Moon, Mars. The general flow of her life as indicated is as follows: The first phase of her life is Venus, which is in conjunction with Mars in the 11th house, not impeded or besieged, but succedant. This looks great, showing a childhood of activity, sport, and a certain wilfulness to her character. The second part of the general flow of her life is shown by the Moon. We could say that emotional dramas, relocations (given that the Moon is in the 1st house), and relationship issues will dominate this period of her life.

The second phase of Nancy's life looks like it might be peppered with issues concerning her physical body, and possibly her home environment. In particular, since the Moon is so prominent, it would be fairly safe to expect a highlighting of issues with her reproductive organs, especially since the Moon rules the 5th house as well. The opposition of the Moon to Uranus might manifest as surgeries on her ovaries, her uterus, her breasts, or her abdomen. As we discussed in Amanda's case, it might also suggest a degree of volatility in ongoing emotional stability.

The Uranus/Pluto conjunction is generational, so the impact of that conjunction is largely collective, and the opposition to the Moon merely highlights her personal experience of collectively emerging infertility issues. Bearing in mind that we are looking at her vitality and general life flow, and remembering that her Sun has accidental dignity and strength in Capricorn and is in the 10th house, the chart does not necessarily indicate poor health or terminal illness. The Sun is the Hyleg and thus gives the chart promise.

Nancy's Almuten of Pregnancy is Jupiter, in detriment in Gemini, angular in the 4th house, Lord of the Chart, and ruler of the MC. Jupiter is also squared by Pluto, Uranus and Saturn, and opposed by Mercury, its dispositor. Basically it is not in good shape, but we can moderate the Uranus/Pluto conjunction opposed to Saturn as a generational marker. Jupiter at the point of the T-square functions in much the same way and, read this way, the outcome for her is not as gloomy as it might at first look. If we remember from Amanda's chart the concept of detriment means being out of the mainstream, applied to fertility potential, we would expect deviance in the age at pregnancy and the means of conceiving, as well as getting pregnant out of wedlock and/or with someone of a different race or cultural group.

Nancy already had two children – the first out of wedlock and the second unexpectedly. Both of these children came in the first phase of her life, i.e. before she turned twenty-eight. She was much younger than her peer group when she had her children and, though their father was of the same culture, he was considerably older than herself and her peer group. All these factors place these conceptions out of the mainstream.

Nancy's Almuten of Pregnancy is Jupiter, in Gemini, which is an air sign. So in her diurnal chart, the first triplicity ruler of her Almuten of Pregnancy is Saturn. Natally, Saturn is angular (just), not in detriment, attended by Jupiter (Lord of the Chart), but opposed by Uranus/Pluto. Saturn sextiles the Sun (rather wide, but valid) and is the ruler of the Sun. Nancy first found herself pregnant at the age of twenty-four and gave birth to a child in the same year. When she conceived, it was a 1st house profected year, ruled by Jupiter, the Almuten of Pregnancy. The first triplicity ruler of the Almuten – Saturn – was operative at the same time that Venus was the triplicity ruler of her Ascendent and her Sun. Venus as triplicity ruler describes a healthy body, lots of vitality, and plenty of passion as expressed in the Mars/Venus conjunction in the 11th (5th of her 7th). So one could assume that this first phase would be good for conception and pregnancy. And indeed it was.

The second triplicity ruler of her Almuten of Pregnancy is Mercury, also in detriment, in the sign of the MC, besieged by Saturn and Uranus/Pluto and opposed by Jupiter, and also disposited by Jupiter. Although in the MC, this placement of Mercury is not particularly dignified, especially since Mercury rules the fallopian tubes in the first place; the applying aspect of Mercury to form the Grand Cross raises some questions as to the ability of Mercury to contribute positively as a triplicity ruler. Nancy had already had two serious operations to her fallopian tubes before this part of her life unfolded; she had her fallopian tubes tied during a challenging marriage, then untied again at the age of thirty-one when she remarried. After several attempts at artificial insemination, and one attempt at IVF, Nancy finally chose to stop, eventually never falling pregnant in the second phase of fertile life.

At the time of the IVF treatment when Nancy and Lisa went in together, Nancy was thirty-eight, so it was a 3rd house profected year, ruled by Venus through the sign of Taurus. Jupiter, her Almuten of Pregnancy, has no voice in terms of aspect or being present in the 3rd house. A profection should always be read together with a solar return chart, but it seems worthwhile to assess with a broad stroke first before doing a solar return for each fertile year of life.

**Lisa**

Lisa had short brown hair, and was neat in figure and form; she was bright, intelligent and loved her life on the farm as a dog breeder. Living a solitary life cut off from neighbours and people in general, she was an avid reader and didn't miss the company. Practical and self-sufficient, down to earth, and brought up in a family atmosphere of common sense and strong morals, she was a contentedly steady partner to her husband. Becoming a mother would, she felt, complete her. Her biography thus far was fairly uneventful, and the Uranus/Pluto opposition to her Sun/Saturn says more about the kind of environment into which she was born than about her personal experience of the darker qualities of Saturn/Pluto.

Here comes the tricky part: is Lisa's chart diurnal or nocturnal? In her chart a decision must be made as to whether we take the Sun or the Moon as the main luminary to direct. There is some debate regarding the position of the Sun on the Descendent, and my approach is to actually consider the light at the time of day at that location – meaning literally going outside and checking whether you could actually see the Sun on the horizon. Solar Fire indicates that the Sun is actually 33' below the horizon. In South Africa the declination is such that the Sun rises and sets with remarkable speed – it seems to shoot up in the sky and drop down very suddenly in the evenings – so the astrologer would have to make a judgement call on whether or not to consider it day time or night time depending on visible conditions. It seems to me to be very close, but I would have to consider this a nocturnal chart, since the Sun would have been just below the horizon.

Since her chart is nocturnal, the sequence of the triplicity rulers of the Moon will then be: Jupiter, Sun, Saturn. We are interested in the second part of her life, which is ruled by the Sun. The Sun is not in detriment. It is angular, conjunct the ruler of the 5th house, and the dispositor of her Venus in the 5th. The Sun also makes an aspect to the Part of Fortune, which is in the MC, conjunct Jupiter, ruler of her Sun. The general flow of the second part of her life looks good to me.

The triplicity rulers of the Ascendant, indicating her health, are in sequence: the Moon, Venus, Mars. Venus claims rulership of this part of her life; Venus is in the 5th house of children and sensuality. She makes a small semi-square (in modern aspect patterning) to Saturn, who receives her from her exaltation. As a broad comment on this part of her life, we might say that children and creativity are a big part of the focus in Lisa's activities for this period, which is encouraging. Lisa's chances of falling pregnant are thus improved in the second phase of her life, her health is good, and her physical body is Venus-orientated.

The Almuten of Pregnancy for Lisa is Mars, in the fire sign of Aries in a nocturnal chart, so the triplicity rulers for her Almuten of Pregnancy are, in sequence, Jupiter, Sun, Saturn. The first part of Lisa's fertile life is ruled by Jupiter in Gemini, angular, in detriment, and in hard aspect to Uranus/Pluto and Saturn. Although Jupiter is conjunct the Part of Fortune, it does seem like a rather unfortunate signature for pregnancy. The second triplicity ruler for her Almuten of Pregnancy is the Sun, which is ruled by Jupiter and is not in detriment. It is angular and with the ruler of her 5th house. The Sun is in Venus' exaltation, with Venus in the fifth, so my feeling is that the second part of her life holds greater potential for children. Also, her age by profection is thirty-seven, and is consequently a '2nd house' year, ruled by her angular Mars which is also her Almuten of Pregnancy, so her chances are thus greatly improved by having treatment at this age. Nancy, who we recall was thirty-eight at the time of treatment, had less luck with profections, as her Almuten of Pregnancy had no voice during her 3rd house profection year, which was ruled by Venus.

**The Gruelling Process of IVF**

IVF treatment involves taking drugs to stimulate the production of eggs, each day for eight consecutive days (depending on the type of hormone used by the specialist). These injections are administered either at home (by a co-operative spouse) or at a nearby clinic (by a nurse or a GP). The drugs are expensive and create such hormonal swings that it is truly a miracle that the spouse (if the male donor) is alive and well enough to provide the much-needed sperm sample some two weeks later. The injections are painful and can wear a person down emotionally. After the specialist has scanned the woman, to see whether she has produced eggs with follicles, a day will be suggested to 'retrieve these eggs' – this is a euphemism for puncturing the internal wall of your vagina, poking a long needle into the nearby ovary, sucking the egg down the tube of the needle and into a test tube, and repeating the process until there are no more eggs. For some women with the Moon in Sagittarius, who have duly produced some twenty eggs, this can be more than a little uncomfortable. The process is usually performed under deep sedation, wherein no pain is felt and no memory of the procedure is remembered. Then the woman usually goes home nursing cramps which settle down to the kind of pain associated with menstruation, and there is some bleeding. After two days, the clinic might call to say that the egg and sperm have fertilised, they might tell you how many embryos are busy 'hatching' and when they would like to see you back to re- implant them. Every situation is different from here on in; some doctors prefer to put back eight-cell embryos, some prefer the embryos to be at the blastocyst stage. Whatever the case, the woman is then required to hop up on the table, with a full bladder, and if she watches the screen carefully, might be able to catch the moment the minute embryo is released from the top of the plastic pipette that is being inserted through her cervix directly into her uterus.[57]

It is preferable that re-implantation is carried out with at least eight-cell embryos, and not fewer, and it is also preferred that they have been self-fertilised. Embryos that are a result of ICSI because of morphology problems in sperm are considered inferior because of possible damage to the egg during the process of imposed fertilisation, and also because of inherent chromosomal defects sometimes present in sperm with morphology problems.[58]

There are different protocols in different countries as to the number of embryos that are re-implanted and the average seems to be three, but in the UK the number is two.[59] In some countries it is possible to re-implant up to five embryos at a time – doctors who do this think that it will increase the chance of a conception. Of course, the reason that conservative regulating bodies recommend three or less embryos at a time is because of the risks associated with multiple births. But many women in their late thirties and early forties, with severe fertility issues, might prefer to gamble and increase their chances of a 'twofer' – as twin births resulting from IVF are now colloquially called. Any birth resulting from IVF, ZIFT, or GIFT is considered precious, and usually the child is delivered by caesarean section under the strict control of the medical profession.[60] It is in the process of choosing the 'best' embryos that doctors are often accused of gender manipulation and tampering with gene material. It is already possible to manipulate gender to some degree, and it will very soon be possible to tamper (legally) with gene material before re-implantation.

After the re-implantation is complete, the woman goes to a ward for a little lie-down and a cup of tea, and is usually allowed home after an hour or so. In 2013, some clinics allowed acupuncture to be practised immediately after implantation in the recovery room, but that is a new development. Ten days after the woman has returned home, she will have a blood test to see whether or not her uterus has accepted the embryos, and whether she has started producing enough pregnancy hormones to register on a test.

## Enter the Fertility Astrologer

As a fertility astrologer, part of the job is to elect time frames for successful implantation of the embryos. This isn't as easy as it sounds, since the time frame given is usually a few days, and it is determined by the cycle of the woman involved, and by the healthy maturation of her eggs and embryos, once fertilised. It is also determined by factors such as public holidays, weekends, and office hours. Once a woman has embarked on a cycle of IVF, it is a process that cannot be altered or changed. This is an expensive procedure, and once started it is not advisable to discontinue unless there is a medical reason to do so. Ideally, the woman will consult the astrologer well before she begins, to establish whether or not it is a good time to do so, or not. I use slow moving planets and transits in my practice to alleviate the stressful task of timing a cycle, so solar arcs and transits of Jupiter are practical to use. Sometimes, however, the client will ask if a specific day is better for implantation, and this is where I have found that fixed stars really come into their own.

### Fixed Stars

As demonstrated with Amanda's chart, fixed stars are invaluable in adding to a narrative, and more so because they are active at certain locations at certain times each year, and every year. So predictions for certain types of activities are sometimes better revealed by stars, while individual reactions/choices are well-articulated through planets in natal charts and their transits. And in this happy collaboration the native often places himself/herself (usually unconsciously) at a location that will best provide the necessary outcome for a particular transit or alignment of planets.

Humans have seemingly always had a dialogue with the night sky.[61] The stars have been our navigational tools, for timing agricultural phases and for inspiring one another with myths and narratives that describe the human condition and the full range of relationship – social, familial, national, global. This perennial relationship with the sky and the alignment of human activity with the rising and setting of constellations demonstrates a conviction that certain places have certain energies at certain times, that there is some collectively-held understanding that there is a preferred time for certain activities at certain locations during the passage of the Sun through the sky during the course of the year. Broadly speaking, it explains why in some cultures there is still a 'season' for marriage, and a season for celebrating the dead, and for ritually recognising both the holy and the unholy. There are times for mourning and times for ploughing, and there are definite seasons for harvest and fertility.

The ancient Greeks had appropriate seasons for all aspects of life, including of course, and pivotally, a season of copulation for reproduction.[62] This timing coincided with the rising and setting of certain stars, most notably the Pleiades and Arcturus. In his studies of the history of sexuality, Michel Foucault discusses a treatise from the Hippocratic collection, called A Regimen for Health:

> Thus the winter regimen should be subdivided as the season itself demands, into a period of forty-four days that extend from the setting of the Pleiades to the Solstice, then into an exactly equivalent period followed by a relaxation of the regimen. Spring begins with a period of thirty-two days, from the rising of Arcturus and the arrival of the swallows to the equinox; within this time span, the season should be divided into six periods of eight days. Then comes the summer season which comprises two phases; from the rising of the Pleiades to the solstice, and from the solstice to the equinox. From that time to the setting of the Pleiades, one should spend forty-eight hours preparing for the 'winter regimen'.[63]

The careful noting of the confluence of natural omens (swallows) and visual astrology (rising and setting of stars, including the constellation of Pisces, formerly known as the Swallows) is indicative of a collective who recognised the holistic nature of the world and who acted in accordance with it. Given the ubiquity of this ancient practice, we just might have a distant cellular memory of the myths connected with the seasons and an accompanying almost-memory of an efficacious link between the seasons and the optimisation of our biological functioning; thus, by bringing this link more fully into consciousness, the astrologer can maximise a client's chances of success by doing the right treatments at the right time of year. I often wonder, as an astrologer, if we humans, as people born to a cultural group at a certain location, really do inherently or subconsciously read and understand the narrative in the sky, and if we respond on some physical or sympathetic level to the movement of the constellations through the sky. Maybe, when we look to the sky, we are prompting our subconscious to thoughts of activity that are entrenched in our mythical memory, and perhaps with good reasons that only become clear when our more modern, 'rational' processes fail us.

### 'Midwife' stars

Some fifty bright stars are relevant for fixed star work, and while far from complete, this collection of significant stars and their constellations – and the myths and narratives that are associated with them – is rich and informative.[64] At least nine stars are, without doubt, linked to fertility, and these stars appear again and again in the charts of the fertility cases I have encountered. Other stars occur with the same regularity in my charts but they are not explicitly described as being fertile. The reason for this could be that writers and observers have most often been people of the northern hemisphere and the sky narrative might look very different to them at different times of the year, and certain stars of the southern hemisphere might never rise or set, and thus may have escaped attention and articulation by astrologers in the past. Until more research has been done on all stars in all locations, both in the northern and southern hemispheres, we cannot create a definitive list of 'fertile stars'. In the meantime, it is useful to look at the ten or so that are already linked with fertility in our cultural myths and legends.

When using fixed stars, just as when we use planets, it is not enough to emphasise one star in delineation, or, on the other hand, to use them all. *Starlight* software will produce a list of parans – relationships that particular stars have with angles and planets – and this list can produce as many as thirty stars to planets; some planets will have seven or more stars in paran and some planets might have none. The relevance of there being no parans to a particular planet only becomes apparent when the astrologer decides to place emphasis on that planet, in terms of whether or not that planet is the chart ruler, the significator, or the Almuten of any particular issue on the table. In that case the absence of a connection becomes meaningful, as we will see.

### 'Diplomat' planets

Stars, by nature, move so slowly that they appear to be static in the sky; they rise and set at the same time, year in and year out, for any given, specific location. Planets move like actors on the starry stage, and interact with the stars by their movement through the constellations; they seemingly wander through narratives and animate the energy of myths through this interaction. It's as if the stars are silent, unable to contribute unless a planet intercedes on our behalf. Brady describes the significance of a star that rises or sets with the Sun as having roughly the energy of that star walking with the mortals on the earth. The type of energy determines what activity is taking place at certain latitudes.

In electional charts it is preferable to choose the appropriate energy for the appropriate activity. In choosing times for treatments, I select groupings of the following stars linked to Mercury, to the angles, and to the Almuten of Pregnancy. I prefer to stress the parans to Mercury, since Mercury signifies the astrologer and the doctor, as well as the fallopian tubes.

### Fertile stars

*Sadalmelek * Sadalsuud * Sirius * Spica * Alkes * Acubens * Alphecca * Capella **

Each of these fertile stars (with the exception of Sadalmelek and Sadalsuud) belong to different constellations and describe fertility narratives that are slightly different in emphasis and essence.

*Sadalmelek* and *Sadalsuud* are found in the constellation of Aquarius; they are considered to be extremely lucky stars and they are found in the river of the water cascading from the amphora of the Great One.[65] These stars are untouchable in terms of fertile potential – they articulate the true potential of creativity, whether one is looking for material wealth, artistic creativity or human reproduction. These stars rise and set as a pair, so they ensure a fairly long 'season' of fertile energy for a location.

*Sirius*, the Dog Star, which heralds the appearance of Orion the Great Hunter in the night sky, is a very bright star and has a rather interesting association with IVF. Sirius has had a long association with the Goddess Isis – this star is seen to be an embodiment of her; more traditionally Isis is linked to the constellation of Virgo, and here we find the correlation between the corn goddess myth and the fertility link with agriculture.[66]

We have already encountered Sirius in Amanda's chart. If you look closer, the narrative of Osiris (later Greek Orion) and Isis is actually somewhat arresting, all the more so when looked at through the lens of modern assisted fertility. In the myth, Seth dismembers the body of Osiris and scatters the parts all over the world; in deep mourning, Isis, together with her sister Nepthys, manage to find and reassemble all of Osiris' body except for the genitalia. Isis fashions a phallus (most likely from a corn cob, since she is the Goddess of Corn) and manages to impregnate herself, thereupon giving birth to Horus. Step aside Louise Brown – there is another contender for the world's first IVF baby!

*Spica* is found in the left hand of the Goddess in the constellation of Virgo – the bright star that signifies the fruits of labour in her hand. This star brings rewards and brilliance to all it touches, and to have this star linked to a fertility electional chart is a good omen. Brady has the following to say about the Goddess of Virgo:

> The early Arabs called her Al Adhra al Nathifah, the Innocent Maiden… To the Greeks she was Demeter, goddess of the harvest, who withdrew herself and her seasons from the earth when Pluto abducted her daughter. They also saw her as Erigone, a maiden who became so distressed at the ways of the human race that she hanged herself. By the time of Christianity she had become Mary holding the Child.[67]

In the creation myths of Venus, Horus, and Jesus Christ, there is no mention of sexual activity – all conceptions were immaculate, all were conceived out of the norm, or with divine intervention. I wonder if this is the (less admissible) reason why some orthodox religions are against IVF – does this method of conception make the human born of IVF equal to the Gods? Is this the hubris – as opposed to the doctors *playing* God?

*Alkes* was once the brightest star of the constellation named The Crater, but has since dimmed. The Crater is depicted in various writings as a vase, a chalice, a cup or container for wine, and Alkes is found at the base of this vessel. An inscription found on an Egyptian vase reads:

> "Wise ancients knew when the Crater rose to sight
> Nile's deluge had attained its height"[68]

The linking of the constellation with the rising of the Nile river is an overt reference to fertility. Other stars (for example, Sirius) that are linked to the seasonal flooding of the Nile, indicate not only agricultural but also human fertility.

In Brady's book *Star and Planet Combinations* the physiological correspondence in natal chart work is given as: 'The ovaries or testes - the quality of one's genetic material.' Brady does not limit the star to human fertility and says that the chalice or cup can be regarded as the 'Well of Apollo', the Holy Grail of the Christian mysteries and a 'vessel that holds life and is therefore sacred.'[69]

*Acubens* is linked with the concept of the 'cradle of humanity' – the Egyptians called this constellation 'Scarab'; later Christian writers would refer to it as the 'Manger' and the two outstretched arms of the constellation are called the 'Aselli' or asses/donkeys. It is in the constellation of Cancer (water triplicity) and, as such, could be a harbinger of rain, and consequent fertility. Brady says:

> This star is linked with the energy of life-giving, the Gateway of life and therefore the concept of resurrection… You may be involved with the bringing in of new life, or with helping in the process of death.[70]

Brady also lists the physiological correspondence as: 'The Reproductive system, the power of generativity, and the future of one's family line.'[71]

*Alphecca* is in the Corona Borealis, and as such has connotations of a crown: royalty, flowers, and thorns. It is a marriage star, and more especially since in my work it is seen to rise a month before Sadalmelek and Sadalsuud, giving a social sequence of marriage and then conception in the traditionally acceptable order. Brady gives a slightly challenging spin on the star, indicating that the gift of the crown comes with a price, and that hardship and difficulties sometimes follow. Her research supports this thinking, but in fertility charts and especially electional ones, I am not so focused on the hardship that might follow, but more anxious to take advantage of the promise of the gift (the baby). This star is a forerunner of the season of Sadalmelek and Sadalsuud and so its appearance increases the length of time that I have to select a good chart.

*Capella* is one of the most difficult stars to come to terms with – the myths are confusing and contradictory. Essentially the constellation

Auriga – The Charioteer – concerns two stories. In one myth, a chariot was built to hide the snake feet of Attica, son of Hephaestus, and to carry him.[72] In the other myth, a goat, or sea-goat, nurses two kids while holding the reins of a chariot. The goat was said to have nursed Zeus and as a token of gratitude was placed in the heavens; the goat also has a connection with the sea-goat associated with the sign of Capricorn.[73] But the most curiously apt weaving of myth in modern times has to be Brady's overlay of an ancient Celtic narrative onto Capella, offering a new synthesis that not only seems to retrospectively make sense of these contradictions, but has proved itself in predictive star work in my fertility charts. In the myth of Macha, she is called upon to compete in a man's race (world) while pregnant with twins. The physical exertion of the race, which she runs as a result of her husband's foolish boast, forces her into labour and she gives birth in the field.[74] This story is about a lack of respect for a woman, especially when pregnant. I think I could take this myth a step closer to the twenty-first century and call it 'Single Mother in the City' – a theme of a woman competing in a man's world while trying to raise children unaided, disrespected, and unacknowledged.

**General supporting stars**
*Regulus * Aldebaran * Rigel * Betelgeuse * Sualocin*

These supportive stars usually operate in the mainstream establishment, ensuring the proper running of administration, the conferring of honours, the quest for justice, and technological breakthroughs.

*Regulus* linked to Mercury can signify a good, honest and talented fertility doctor, or a morally prudent astrologer, or a particularly careful and studious lab technician who thaws out the embryos on the day of treatment. This star seems to endorse the activities of the day when it is the heliacal rising star and can help overcome some really difficult situations as long as one seeks to do the right thing and avoids intrigue.

*Aldebaran* seems to endorse the legal position, having to do with maintaining the status quo, but if help is sought, and if the request is for something honourable and legally entitled, support will be found, if this star is linked to the electional chart.

*Rigel* seems to indicate that as long as the motivation or the request for help is linked somehow to gaining knowledge, then support is assured.

Sometimes it presents in fertility charts where things are not quite straightforward and new techniques, astrological or medical, are learned or tested in the process.

*Betelgeuse* – Brady says of this star: 'This is one of the great stars of the sky and can talk of unbridled success without complications'.[75] It is often present where physical agility or talent is successful; whatever complicated procedure is to be undertaken is supported by the presence of this star.

*Sualocin* seems to indicate the desire of the technicians, or the astrologer, to stretch their technology just for its own sake – either to test it or to prove something to themselves. While generally supportive, it is a gentle star; it doesn't have the supreme powers required to overcome really challenging charts. It can seduce you with the playfulness of technique, so be wary lest you lose the focus you need.

### Difficult or tricky stars
*Algol * Capulus * Facies * Alphard * Antares*

Stars that often accompany fertility treatment sometimes articulate the difficult energies that are involved in such treatments, and should not been seen as a wholly negative influence, but rather a description of the circumstances, especially the anguish and pain, involved in undertaking IVF and other invasive procedures. Of course these difficult stars have the potential to wreak havoc with attempts to conceive, but as always with astrological delineation, no single signature should form the basis of a judgement.

*Algol* and *Capulus* are a pair of stars that sometimes describe the pain and anguish, the bloody trials, and the female fury that accompanies invasive procedures like IVF. Capulus with emphasised planets, such as the Moon or the Almuten of Pregnancy, proves to have a negative impact on charts; it is best to avoid it. Algol seems to be more descriptive of the event, and my recent thinking is that Algol carries the energy of the Greek Furies (think pro-lifers), who are omnipresent at events where family blood is spilt.

*Facies* does not normally present with problems in fertility electional charts; it seems to give the chart an intense focus, and a competitive edge. Ruthless decisions have to be made, and this energy is required to make them. Facies can promise a positive outcome – one of the lighter interpretations for this otherwise nasty star is that of prophecy, and if the client is practising some sort of divination, omen reading or astrology, then the predictive quality of the moment is intense and focused on success.

*Alphard* is like an eclipse during a hijacking, a wrong turn in a wrong neighbourhood. Visually Alphard is in the constellation Hydra opposite the constellation of Leo, and separated by the ecliptic – really on the wrong side of town. This star can point to hidden and unrealised emotions connected with the activity that you are doing, and in fertility work it can bring loss as a result of unresolved issues to do with nurturing and child rearing, or unspoken fears of pregnancy, or perceived loss of sexuality within the relationship, that have not been addressed.

*Antares* gives any electional chart an obsessional quality, sometimes to the detriment of those involved; health issues can be ignored in the attempt to try yet another IVF cycle. Fractured energy concentrated in short intense bursts is not conducive to conception, so one has to watch that moderation is practised, and that the intensity of this star is managed. These aren't the only stars I use, but they are the most common across my fertility electional charts.

**Technical note on use of Parans in *Starlight***

If you open a chart in *Starlight* and click the *double text* button on the top menu, you will find the option to view both the Mundane Parans and the Daily Parans of that day. They are different.

The Mundane Parans is a list of parans to planets for the moment that a particular star became the heliacal rising star for that period.[73] This marks a period of time – from the couple of days to sometimes two weeks that this star has 'rulership' – much like a chart ruler. This heliacal rising star and all the planetary parans set the tone for the kind of activity that will be taking place at that particular latitude or location.

In the Daily Parans, the list will be the most recent list of parans to planets; the heliacal rising or setting will remain the same and you might pick up some stars on the angles of the chart for that moment/day that are different from the Mundane Parans list. These changes are to be seen in the context of the Mundane Parans, but are more informative of subtler energy changes that have occurred on that particular day. As a memory aid, it may be useful to think of the Mundane list as being the natal chart and the Daily list to be a progression chart – not literally, of course, just metaphorically.

**Location Matters: A Place to Conceive**
Given that parans are determined by the location where the chart is being cast, it goes without saying that the location of the attempts at conception should always be taken into account. Nancy and Lisa went in for their embryo transfer on 16 February 2004, in Cape Town, South Africa. It was a sunny day, around 26 degrees, and high summer. Sadalsuud had become the heliacal rising star just the day before, and the women would have started their drug treatments on 5 February 2004, when Acubens was the heliacal setting star. (There are subtle differences between heliacal rising or setting, but not enough research has been done to articulate just what these differences could be – suffice to say that when the star is seen on the horizon, its energy suffuses the location through the contact of being either rising or setting). So, right from the start, this looked like the combination of a perfect time and a perfect place.

**Transits**
Let's examine the transits active for Lisa and Nancy. For 16 February 2004, Lisa enjoyed the traditionally fertile transit of Jupiter to a luminary, her Sun, by applying opposition, but before it opposed her Sun, the greater benefic also aspected her Moon, the Uranus/Pluto conjunction, her Part of Fortune, Saturn and then the Ascendant and her natal Jupiter. Whew! How can one not get pregnant with those transits? For Nancy, 16 February 2004 brought Jupiter into opposition to with her Saturn (just past). It then squared her Mercury, applied to oppose her Moon, conjoin her Uranus/Pluto conjunction, and conjunct her Descendant, before squaring her natal 4th house Jupiter.

In both charts, the transiting Moon-Saturn opposition stretched across the 10th/4th axis, with Nancy's chart looking a bit disappointing considering Saturn was by whole sign in the 5th house and is not the Almuten of Pregnancy, and therefore could only bring limitations and obstacles to the party. But, in Nancy's favour, she has already proven capable of falling pregnant and delivering healthy children, in spite of a natal Moon/Saturn conjunction. Recall that her Almuten of Pregnancy is Jupiter, which is the Lord of her Chart, her MC and her Moon/Saturn conjunction. However, it is in detriment, both natally and by transit.

In Lisa's chart Saturn is the ruler of the 5th house, dispositor of her 5th house Venus, and is opposing the Moon in the sign of the 5th. Altogether a much better arrangement. Lisa's Almuten of Pregnancy is Mars transiting Venus' sign of Taurus, squaring her 5th house Venus, and she is in a Mars profected year. Mars in her natal chart is strong, angular and in rulership, but the transiting Mars is in detriment, so a non-mainstream pregnancy is more likely than a natural one.

**Facing Medical/Physical Reality**
Nancy managed to produce eight beautiful eggs, four of which fertilised with her husband's healthy sperm by themselves, and the other four were fertilised using ICSI. On the day of implantation, these eggs were eight-cell embryos, good looking and going places. Lisa only managed to produce two eggs, and by the time they were re-implanted in her uterus, they had only matured into one four-cell embryo and one single cell embryo. Lisa chose to continue with her treatment after such disappointing maturation of these embryos because this was likely to be the last treatment she and her husband could afford and the last chance they had of ever becoming parents.

The medical consensus would support that Nancy stood the better chance of becoming pregnant because of her previous history of successful births and the advanced and established maturation of her embryos, while Lisa was severely disadvantaged with only two embryos to choose from, neither looking encouraging, and in previous treatments she had produced better looking embryos and still not succeeded. The same fertility specialist performed the same procedure on both women just minutes apart; the same lab technician and nurse were on duty; and both women returned to the ward to lie down for the same amount of time before going home. As we just observed, both were having a transit of Jupiter to the luminaries, in Lisa's case to both her Sun and Moon and angles, in Nancy's to her Moon and angles. They were virtually the same age, height and weight, both in enviable health and full of vitality.

Given the profound similarities, let's recap the astrological differences. Nancy is in the second phase of her fertile life, which means the Moon (not in a good condition natally) is the ruler of the general flow, and Mars (fair condition) is the ruler of her health. Lisa is also in the second phase of her life, the ruler of the general flow of it is Venus (in the 5th, not besieged or afflicted), and the ruler of her health is also Venus. Lisa's profected year is ruled by her Almuten of Pregnancy, Mars, strongly placed in rulership, while Nancy's profected ruler is Venus, conjunct malefic Mars disposited by Saturn.

In Nancy's favour is her history of fertile success and if we look at the last time she conceived, she had chosen a remarkably similar season for trying to get pregnant. A full Jupiter cycle previously, almost to the day, Nancy had conceived her second child, under a transit of Jupiter in Virgo, aspecting her mutable grand cross and angles in much the same way. (See Figure 4.3)

**Nancy's Previous Conception**
Furthermore, Nancy had conceived this child in spite of a transit of Saturn to her natal Venus/Mars conjunction in the 11th house (5th of her husband). She would have been in the first phase of her life – with both the general flow and her health being ruled by Venus. She was twenty-seven years old at the time and her profected 4th house year was ruled by Mercury, containing her Almuten of Pregnancy, and aspected by it natally. An interesting point to notice is that the Moon in the conception chart is applying to a conjunction of Saturn, and this was a successful conception – transits of Saturn to natal Venus, or a Moon/Saturn conjunction in conception or electional charts, are not always contra-indicators of success. Nancy therefore had no reason to believe that her attempt to get pregnant a second time on similar transits was going to be any different.

The only other difference in comparing Nancy's previous conception with the current attempt, is that of course the first successful conception was with her first husband and the second attempt is with a second husband. This is not to be underestimated in terms of fertility astrology. Both charts work together; in some cases the man's chart can outweigh the woman's in terms of essential dignity and power of transit, in other cases the reverse is true. Sometimes clients with heavy 11th house planets choose a partner who seems to want or need children more than they do, and they co-operate with the process for other benefits and needs that are served by the relationship.

70    Fertility Astrology

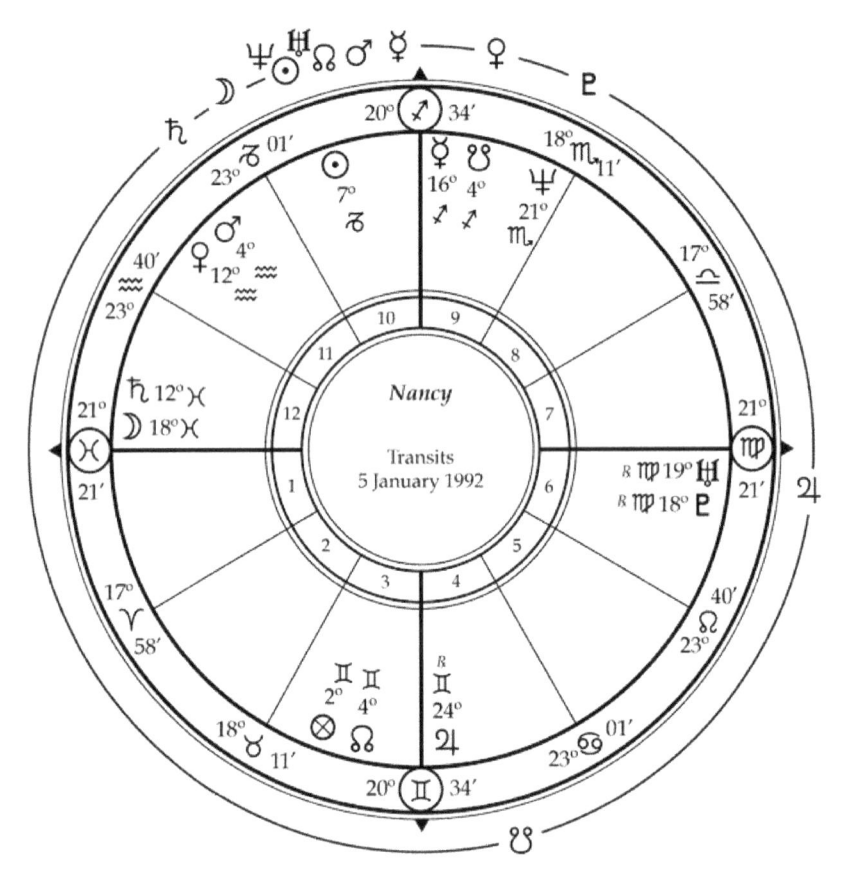

Figure 4.3: Nancy's previous conception

**The Remarkable Outcome**
On 26 February 2004, Nancy learned that she was not going to be a mother for a third time, while on their farm, Lisa and her husband quietly celebrated the miracle of a conception against all expectation. So, why did Nancy not fall pregnant while Lisa did? They both had Jupiter aspecting luminaries, they were almost the same age, they had almost identical chart angles; how did one achieve success and not the other? And does astrology have an adequate answer to that question?

Although the triplicity rulership (of life phase and Almuten of Pregnancy) supports the outcome, and profections and solar returns are richly descriptive, a modern astrologer would have had a hard time delineating the disparity without the use of medieval technique. So what other tools do we astrologers have to help with predictive work? In the effort to provide answers for my clients, I have turned to fixed stars.

On the day of the embryo transplant, the Mundane Parans (which ruled that particular time period) showed that Sadalsuud was the heliacal rising star – indicating immense fertile energy. These women chose a good day to have this procedure. When Sadalsuud is the heliacal rising star, Brady says that it indicates 'a fortunate event, a lucky chance'. Acubens was the heliacal setting star, which brings up, 'questions and issues around the sacredness of life'. The Sun also had star parans for that day: it was 'rising when Sadalsuud is Rising' which indicates that 'after a drought comes rain, literally or metaphorically' and also 'setting when Antares is on Nadir' indicating 'an obsessive person'.[77]

Mercury – the signifier for the doctor, the astrologer, and the fallopian tubes – had in paran for that day:

*Rising when Arcturus is Culminating* [...]
    A new invention, a bright idea
*Rising when Altair is Rising* [...]
    Military ideas and people take centre stage
*Culminating when Mirach is Rising* [...]
    The mediator, finding the middle ground

When looking at the mundane parans, it's useful to check if the planet that serves as the client's Almuten of Pregnancy is making parans with any stars at that location. To be clear, this is not the natal placement of the client's own Almuten. So we are looking at whether the transiting planet is making parans; and it is the resonance between the parans of the transiting planet and this planet's role as the client's Almuten of Pregnancy that forms the key link.

So for Lisa, whose Almuten of Pregnancy is Mars, we find that transiting Mars for this day was in paran with Procyon (setting when Procyon is culminating), which indicates 'A rash or violent act, or a sudden breakthrough achievement'. However, for Nancy, whose Almuten of Pregnancy is Jupiter, we find *no parans to any stars* for this location on this day whatsoever to transiting Jupiter.

Looking at the daily parans for a deeper and richer informative take on the mundane chart, I note that the fertile star Spica culminated on one of the angles of the daily parans, which Brady says, among other things, has 'a gift that can bring joy to others'. This was a fertile location on that day! The Moon, Mercury and Mars (Lisa's Almuten of Pregnancy!), all made significant parans, however there were no parans with Jupiter (Nancy's Almuten of Pregnancy). As Jupiter wandered through the constellations, it wasn't actually on the stage that day as it didn't form a relationship with a star. Jupiter had no voice; it couldn't intercede on Nancy's behalf on *that* day at *that* location. No pregnancy appeared possible.

One can increase the orbs used with fixed stars to increase the chances of picking up a star paran, but I am wary of doing so arbitrarily, as it can be as distorting as disregarding planetary orbs, or house cusps. Sometimes I increase them as a matter of interest to see how close the planet is to being in paran to another star, and what type of energy is closest to hand. Considering this, if the orb of Jupiter is increased to 4 degrees instead of the standard 2 degrees, parans are made with Bellatrix, El Nath, and Zosma, but none of these stars are 'fertile stars'. At the end of the day, and stretching the lens as much as I dared, there were still no fertile stars to be found with Jupiter. For Nancy, this was not to be a time for babies.

**Notes**

56. For Roe v. Wade see: https://www.law.cornell.edu/supremecourt/text/410/113 [Accessed April 4, 2017]; for the history of reproduction, see Kay Elder, Doris J. Baker, and Julie A. Ribes, *Infections, Infertility, and Assisted Reproduction*, p.7.
57. Blastocyst – see Glossary.
58. ICSI – see Glossary.
59. http://www.hfea.gov.uk/2587.html
60. IVF, ZIFT, GIFT– see Glossary.
61. For a history of this period of astronomical and astrological lore see Campion, Nicholas. *The Dawn of Astrology.*
62. The Hippocrates/Galen's Regimen.
63. Foucault, M. and Hurley, R. *The History of Sexuality: The Use of Pleasure*, Vol. 2. p111.
64. *Starlight.*
65. *Fixed Stars*, p.308
66. (http://www.crystalinks.com/sirius.html); *Starlight* [Constellation Virgo].
67. *Fixed Stars*, p.270.
68. Jobes, Gertrude and James. *Outer Space: Myths, Name Meanings, Calendars.*
69. Brady, Bernadette. *Star and Planet Combinations*, p.103.
70. *Fixed Stars*, p.257.

71. *Star and Planet Combinations,* p.74.
72. *Outer Space: Myths, Name Meanings, Calendars,* p.126.
73. Ibid, p.312.
74. *Fixed Stars,* p.70.
75. Ibid, p.168.
76. Heliacal rising star – Glossary
77. All quotes here from *Starlight* delineations.

# 5
# Case Study – Raylene and Jacques
## A Couple in Consultation

So far we have considered the woman's chart in isolation with respect to her fertility, however a partner's chart often plays an extensive role. In the following case study I track a husband and wife, although one could also apply this technique to any couple. The crux here is on who carries the child to term. For example, with lesbian couples, one partner is likely to physically carry the baby, while the other is going to become a parent, and so astrologically, the charts need to be considered in terms of roles. The sperm donor is irrelevant, as his contribution is just that, no commitment, financial or otherwise, so his chart is not part of the family picture. Even if, for some reason, a best friend, or brother is going to donate, it is still not taken into account. However, the chart of a gestational carrier is very important. Her health, her ability to conceive, and so on, are vital to the process, so her chart should be considered, alongside the couple's charts as they are going to become parents, and this will be indicated in the chart. Now let us meet Raylene and Jacques.

**Background**
Raylene met Jacques when they were both nineteen years old and at university together. He proposed to her when she was twenty-four and they decided to try to conceive straight away. As a consequence of recurring teenage acne, Raylene had been on the contraceptive pill 'Diane', since the age of thirteen. She was justifiably concerned about her fertility, but during the months leading up to the wedding, her acne returned and she starting taking the pill again until after the ceremony in June 2005. In June 2006 they started trying a little more seriously to conceive. Raylene came off the pill and started taking herbal supplements, and they tracked her cycle and ovulation, noting that she had a disturbing sixty-day cycle. This was the first indicator of problems to come. In March 2007, Jacques had a sperm test at a fertility clinic. The results were devastating: a low

count and zero morphology. Raylene was diagnosed at the same clinic with PCOS and, at twenty-six years old, they faced the possibility of never becoming parents.

The clinic advised two cycles of IUI (artificial insemination). During these cycles Raylene needed a lot of medication to stimulate her to ovulate. Her hormonal challenges meant that even after a cycle of IVF, the embryos that were harvested were all of an inadequate quality to re-implant. It seemed as though the sperm was a major contributing factor, although at this point no genetic testing had been done to confirm whether it was a sperm or egg issue. The doctors were of the opinion that it was a bit of both – poor egg quality due to the PCOS and poor sperm, resulting in substandard embryos. In short, both partners had fertility problems, and together they compounded the problem.

In April 2008 Raylene had another cycle of IVF. This time she did fall pregnant – there was a heartbeat at six weeks, but sadly, she miscarried at eight weeks. Again, the opinion of the medical team placed the blame on the quality of her eggs and his sperm. Another cycle in August 2008 yielded fifteen eggs but no embryos, again the doctors blamed her egg quality. A further IVF using GIFT (where the embryo is put into the fallopian tube and not directly into the uterus) in December 2008 resulted in more disappointment. The medical team then had the tough conversation about using donor egg and sperm with a couple who were only in their twenties, and who were desperate to be parents.

Jacques was not keen on using donor sperm at all. Raylene pushed for it, following her primal urge to be a mother. Irrational, not sleeping and not always hormonally balanced, she went from one treatment to another, trying some fairly unorthodox methods to get pregnant.

In June 2009, September 2009, and December 2009 the couple experienced more attempts that did not result in pregnancy. With Raylene considering suicide and finding it impossible to go on in this state, she contacted Tertia Albertyn who had an egg donor company in Cape Town. Here she found a compassionate listener and also someone who had my contact details. Raylene wasted no time and made an appointment to see me.

On first review of their charts, although Jacques' sperm issues were fairly obvious to me, Raylene's chart didn't seem as bad as her story reflected. This is the testing point for the astrologer: you hear a really difficult narrative history, then you see a challenged chart, but not nearly as bad as the story suggests. What do you do? Do you go with the story the client and the medical fraternity are telling you, or do you fly with the astrology? Fortunately for me, I had seen a lot of charts by the time I saw Raylene, and I was able to draw on my experience in my practice.

I judged the charts as being the most heartbreaking narratives I had heard thus far, but although Jacques's chart was technically and astrologically more challenging, Raylene's chart was not saying quite the same thing.

**Raylene's chart**

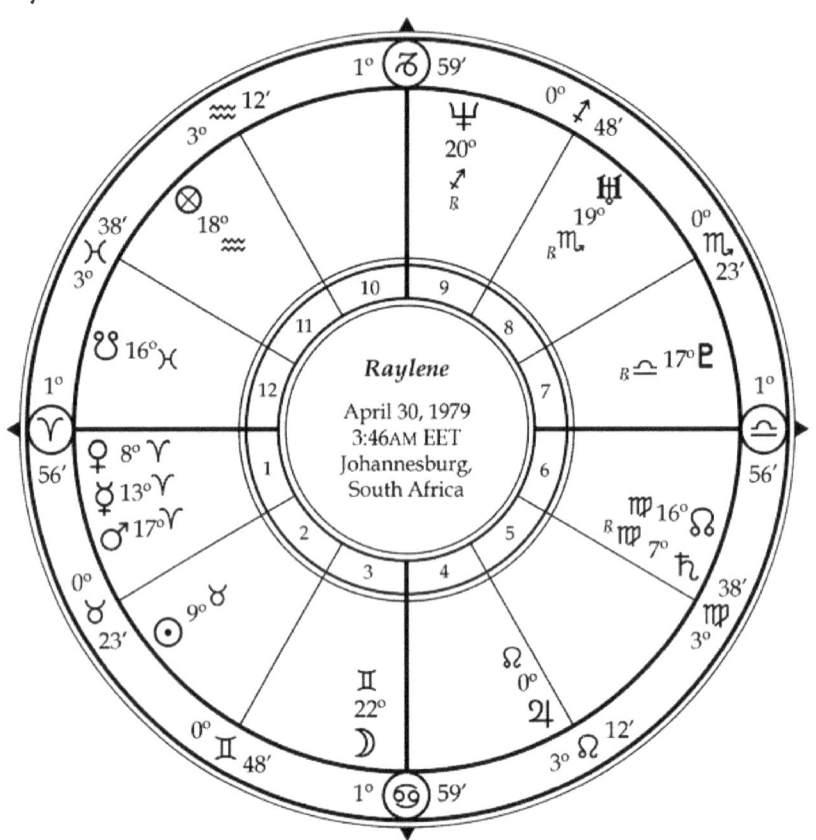

Figure 5.1: Raylene's Chart

In analysing Raylene's chart (Figure 5.1), the Almuten of Pregnancy, the Sun, leaps out at me. It is in Taurus, in the 2nd house, succedent, and seemingly without besiegement. The Sun also indicates a stubborn physicality through the sign of Taurus, so her menstrual cycles are most probably regular, but ovulation can still be variable, and being a Taurean, more than the normal dose of medication might be required to stimulate hormones. Equally, Taureans often suffer from thyroid issues, so this is something to ask about first.

Her fallopian tubes are indicated by Mercury in Aries, conjunct Mars and Venus, all opposite Pluto in Libra in the 7th house. A fire-sign Mercury can indicate ectopic pregnancies, the conjunction to Mars can indicate surgery to the tubes, and the opposition to Pluto is a strong signature for an invasive surgery to tubes, and the destruction of one or both tubes due to inflammation or infection. The only mitigating factor is the conjunction of Mercury with Venus and the fact that Mercury joys in the 1st house. If it were not for those placements, I might conclude that her fallopian tubes are not in the best shape. Her uterus – indicated by the 1st house and its ruler Mars, which is opposite Pluto – is also not looking good. Endometriosis could play a role here, or there could be something wrong with her endometrial lining, and as we know, the blood wall of the uterus is important for implantation. Heavy bleeding during menstruation is also probable. But Mars is in rulership, so we wait to diagnose and look for further information.

Her Moon in Gemini indicates eggs that mature a little out of sync compared to the norm, usually late maturation, as Gemini is also one of the barren signs. On investigation, her eggs might not have a follicle in them, and this might prove tricky on egg retrieval in the process of IVF. The Moon is also opposite Neptune, so sometimes the egg is not physically visible on ultrasound scans. Or the egg can present as perfect and then be found to be subnormal after retrieval. Or there might be some chromosomal damage to the egg, in which case implantation might occur but at some stage there might be arrested development of cell division, and the embryo might not mature into a blastocyst. Frequent miscarriages without any identifiable reason are often attributed to chromosomal defects in the embryo or problems with the lining of the uterus and implantation.

The Moon opposite Neptune also speaks of hormonal imbalance.

78    Fertility Astrology

This may manifest independently and indicate issues during puberty or menopause and have nothing to do with fertility, or it may have a direct bearing on someone's fertility. It may allude to thyroid issues or even be a manifestation of using hormone therapy during aggressive fertility treatment. Sometimes astrologers think of Neptune as a planet of disillusion or illusion, so it is worth noting that the condition of the egg is not what it seems and that sometimes test results can 'lie' and that sometimes perfect looking eggs fail to deliver. As a fertility astrologer you cannot always tell which way it will go, except to say that if other factors point to illusion, then you might need to downplay a positive outcome. Whichever way you view the Moon/Neptune opposition, it offers little relief to Raylene's chart.

**The Triplicity Phase Rulers**
The triplicity phase rulers of her Ascendant, which is in Aries, a fire sign, are: 1) Jupiter, 2) Sun 3) Saturn. Remember, the order of the first two rulers is switched to reflect her night chart. We are really interested in the second phase of her life, beginning on average around age thirty, so we examine the second ruler. The Sun is her Almuten of Pregnancy! So we can say that this is the phase during which she will most likely conceive, which is generic considering most women conceive in this phase, i.e. twenty-five to forty-five years of age. But it is important to understand that now the Almuten of Pregnancy has emphasis. Pay attention to that.

Let's look at the triplicity rulers of her Almuten of Pregnancy. The Sun is in Taurus, an earth sign, and she has a night chart, so the rulers are: 1) Moon, 2) Venus 3) Mars. Again, we are interested in the second phase only, so we examine Venus. Looking at her natal chart, we see that Venus is angular, but in detriment, opposite Pluto, and sextile her Sun (Almuten of Pregnancy). So our initial conclusion could be that yes, it is most likely that she will be pregnant (Venus sextile Sun) but that there will be trauma (Pluto) and opposition and Mars-like surgery.

Then, calculate the triplicity rulers of her main luminary, which in a night chart is the Moon. Her Moon is in Gemini, an air sign, giving us: 1) Mercury, 2) Saturn 3) Jupiter. Looking to Saturn, then, which is the second phase ruler of her overall life circumstance and sense of vitality, we see that Saturn is cadent, in Virgo so no particular strength or dignity, and conjunct the nodal axis, indicating a difficult time in her life. Health issues are going to impact her quality of life. In a modern interpretation, there seems to be a certain compulsion or karmic quality to the conjunction with the nodes. In a medieval interpretation, it looks like this phase of her life is blighted by the conjunction to the nodes.

A summary of the triplicity rulerships could be that the second part of her life is going to be taken up with trying to conceive, experiencing difficulties, surgery and/or disappointment, damage to her fallopian tubes, but eventually some success? I use the question mark because by the time we see her husband's chart it looks very unlikely this couple can have children.

**Returning to Raylene's chart**
Raylene consulted with me in 2009, and in that December she underwent another cycle of donor egg share with IVF which didn't work for either party. My prediction was that April 2010 was auspicious as there was a MC sextile her Venus/Jupiter midpoint by solar arc on 20 April. Solar arcs are quite powerful and they have a long 'hangover' period during which they are still effective. I usually consider the effect of the solar arc to be for three weeks after the exact date, and sometimes for three months in a more diluted fashion.

Raylene and her husband also decided to change clinics after the December 2009 cycle didn't work out. This can be very useful, as a new clinic often retests everything, and the specialist looks with 'new eyes'. In this case, the specialist did pick up that Raylene's FSH indicator was actually within the range of normal and that she didn't have any cysts present due to her previous diagnosis of PCOS. These medical reassurances encouraged them to do the treatment with their own eggs and sperm. The transfer date for the eggs was 3 May 2010, the start date of the treatment would have been 19 April 2010, exactly on the first solar arc of 20 April. The transfer date was as close as possible to the 27 April solar arc. Raylene had this response to my prediction:

> When Nicky advised us to use our own gametes in April 2010 I was skeptical but with six failed IVFs behind us, two of them being donor egg cycles, I was desperate enough to try anything, even returning to what I thought were my poor quality eggs. It was with a mixture of fear and relief that we decided to go ahead with my eggs – fear that we

might just be pouring more money into the bottomless pit and relief that maybe, just maybe, we could conceive with my eggs.[78]

When I asked her afterwards if she believed the astrology, she said:

> Put it this way I didn't believe it would work because of all the past failures, but I had no reason to doubt what you were saying, and I had nothing to lose by using your advice and waiting to try in that specific time. I was hopeful it would work, and I wanted so badly to believe you, but its hard to actually believe it would work. I think you would be a fool to blindly believe. I had to protect myself somehow.[79]

One of the things I look for in chart prediction is that the Almuten of Pregnancy is emphasised by solar arc, transit or profection. Jupiter by transit was applying to her Ascendant by 7 degrees, trining her natal Jupiter on the 5th house Leo (ruled by Almuten of Pregnancy) cusp. In the profected chart, Venus rules the 5th house through the sign of Taurus. Her natal Sun (Almuten of Pregnancy) is in Taurus.

By profection from the Ascendant, Raylene was thirty, which means she was going to be engaged in activities related to the natal 7th house ruled by Venus. Venus natally is in the 1st, conjunct Mars opposite Pluto. This thirtieth year of life was going to be difficult – lots of blood, sweat, and tears literally, and effectively in the house of relationship – not an easy time. As Venus is in the 1st house natally, it suggests also a year of health issues, and changes to her living environment.[80] In conclusion, this is a fertility phase ruled by Venus, and her Almuten of Pregnancy is the Sun, so these two planets need to configure closely in order to make a prediction of pregnancy likely or possible. We also need the blessings of Jupiter, by transit, solar arc, or profection.

**IVF results**

On 19 May 2010, after the implantation of three embryos using their own eggs and sperm, Raylene tested for a positive beta result – it was a decisive positive. But the relevant fertile solar arc (MC sextile Asc) didn't happen until 29 May. Sometimes, due to long hormonal cycles or to the time constraints of the clinic or the doctor, it isn't possible to do the treatments at the exact time of the astrological signatures. For this reason I use solar arcs and transits from slow-moving Jupiter, so that the 'effect' is long lasting, and there is a bigger window of time to work with than using the transit of, say, the Moon. Also, given that there are only two or three really fertile moments in a chart each year, then if you are a couple of weeks out in the start time of your treatment, this is not as much of a problem as you might think. We are also having to match two charts which can be tricky. In this case, Jacques' chart had a potent solar arc on 27 April 2010. This solar arc (Venus conjunct Sun) happened as Raylene started her cycle of injections to prepare for the IVF, and since it has a long influence, being a solar arc, it covered the period to the end of June. Three embryos were implanted, all three took. Raylene decided to keep all of them and didn't go for the recommended 'reduction'. Reduction is when the doctor safely removes one or more of the embryos so as to ensure a safer pregnancy and a live birth. It was very risky to keep all three, but after seven rounds of fertility treatment, she didn't want to take any chances.

On 10 December 2010 Raylene delivered triplets at thirty-three weeks, all healthy, and all have turned into very beautiful little girls. Naturally, the doctors who had thought all along that her egg quality was inadequate had to rethink their judgements. Her astrology at the forty-week mark of her pregnancy was equally relevant. Her due date would have been 2 February 2011, the day Jupiter conjoined her Ascendant, exactly. When looking for potentially fertile times it is useful to look forty weeks ahead and see what is happening astrologically that can support the narrative of a happy ending with a live birth. When one sees that a forty-week period is 'bookended' with two fertility signatures, then one can start being bolder with the prediction. In astrology, fertility signatures can be either a conception or a birth, so one can use the 'end time' as a start time. So if Raylene had still not fallen pregnant by 2 February 2011, she could have used that potentially fertile time to start a treatment.

In hindsight, one of the reasons I think this cycle was successful is that I supported Raylene's own thinking and belief that her eggs were fine. She had resisted the diagnosis of faulty eggs all along, and I had the astrological means to support this. It was as if I had seen through all the medical misdiagnosis and finally 'seen' her and her good eggs. This resonance is reminiscent of Rita Charon and her thinking in *Narrative Medicine*. This pivotal moment of exchange needs to happen in order for the patient to fully open up to the next phase of the healing, that is, the taking charge of one's situation and making a move towards a future goal. I would like to add here that it is not usual for me to want to contradict the medical practitioner at any point without very good reason. I appreciate the trust relationships that patients have with their care-givers and do not seek to disturb that sacred space just so I can score points. However, if I am to be truly professional and have confidence in the astrology that I practise, every now and again I have to point out something I see in the chart that might contradict the current medical opinion. When such a contradiction occurs, I tend to defer to the medical test result. But if there is no conclusive medical result, and no successful pregnancy then I am obliged to voice my professional concerns, and with consideration for the awkward situation it places my client in. I have found that most clients don't tell their partners that they are seeking advice from an astrologer on something as serious as this; many will feel shy admitting it to a medical practitioner, and most definitely feel awkward about contradicting medical advice on the advice of an astrologer, so it behoves the astrologer to proceed with extreme caution in order to avoid upsetting the supportive team who are all trying to achieve the same goal.

**Reading Male Charts for Fertility**
Let's turn now to how to delineate a male chart in fertility. Gender differences in delineation are to be expected, as men respond differently to the prospect of becoming a parent. So in looking at male charts, I find it useful to comment on or ask about the relationships at home when the man was growing up and to what extent he fears repeating the patterning of the past in the future.

Moon/Saturn aspects will be manifested in concerns related to cost of fertility treatments, ability to afford a child, whether they have the time to devoted to the task of raising the child. Sometimes, men have a problem imagining that they will have enough love or nurturing energy required to be a father. I know a lot of clients who are desperately in love with their wives, but worry that a child will upset their relationship and that they don't have the capacity to take on another emotional relationship. Of course once the baby is there, that glorious unending conditional love completely overwhelms them, and they can't understand where that idea came from, but the child as a concept and not a physical reality tends to be a totally different thing.

Men with Venus/Pluto aspects tend to worry about losing the sexual intimacy that they have with their partner. They invest a lot in the sexual relationship and are nurtured by this intimacy, so 'competing' with a breastfeeding baby is something to fear. Uranus/Moon aspects need the freedom to carry on a bachelor lifestyle, keeping independence and hobbies intact, even though their partner is at home with a newborn.

Moon/Neptune men idealise the process of child-raising, comparing their partners to their 'perfect' mothers. Sometimes they even keep the child-raising in the realm of fantasy by always talking about it in future terms, but never actually having a child.

Men with Moon/Mars have the hardest time, since this is one signature that often produces physical as well as psychological manifestations. This signature may attract 'angry women' into the life of the man in question. Angry, competitive women, women who emasculate, women who challenge – these women figures can start off as being mothers who, by accident, find their boy masturbating and who by just a twitch of an eyebrow can leave the boy to understand that what he did was disgusting and shameful or something that 'we don't talk about'. As this boy grows up he might have successful relationships with girlfriends and all is fine until he marries, and his wife would like a child, a male child perhaps. The repressed feelings from childhood emerge. He imagines his partner will 'become' his mother, and he suddenly feels shameful all over again while masturbating in a cup in a doctor's room while trying to conceive through IVF.

The physical manifestation is often in the morphology of the sperm. Sperm has three important criteria – shape or morphology, count, and motility. Morphology is important as the head of the sperm has to release a hormone that weakens the lining of the egg to faciliate the fertilisation of the egg – think of this as a 'May I come in?', a doffing of the hat to the egg.

Men who have been surrounded by angry women often do not feel that polite respect for them. They are angry back, their chivalry has been suppressed, and they don't want to engage with proper respect or gentility. I would say most men with this signature are simply unaware of their feelings. They are not all misogynists (a small percentage might be), they are often just slightly damaged by the impact of such a mother figure.

Since sperm is reproduced every seventy-two days, a psychological shift or change in the way a man feels about these issues may indeed change the nature of the next batch of fresh sperm. Similarly, men with fears about not being a 'good enough' parent can be reassured just by talking to someone sympathetic, and this person could be an astrologer, or it might be a psychologist. It is sometimes hard to engage with conventional therapy at the same time as undergoing IVF treatment. Therapy takes a long time, and IVF can bring out the very worst in people; they can be very vulnerable and might need to concentrate on one thing at a time.

Having medical intervention to achieve conception is tricky for a couple, as there are bound to be issues around blame. Whose fault is it that they're not pregnant? Could it be hers since she had that STI that blocked her tubes, or could it be his since his sperm health has been compromised due to lifestyle choices? For most men, just having their sperm tested is a humiliation, and to be called 'average' is a cruel blow to their manhood. The thought of egg donation is hard enough, but for the average man the concept of using another man's sperm is, well, inconceivable.

The process of having IVF is tough on both parties, but the man plays a more passive role. He stands by and watches while she has to inject herself every day, wincing as the bruises form. Then he must watch while another person scans her vaginally to see if she is ovulating. Finally he is expected to hold his partner's hand while an embryologist and an IVF specialist insert precious embryos into her uterus without sedation. When a cycle of IVF fails, it is usually the male partner who wants to give up first, not because he wants a child any less, but because he can't handle watching someone he loves going through so much medical trauma. I often counsel women to leave the men in the waiting room, to close the bathroom door when injecting, because for the most part, women can handle much more pain and discomfort than men, and it doesn't serve them if their counterpart and teammate gets squeamish and then chickens out of the next cycle. It is better to keep it together, keep strong and go another round.

In a male chart, we are concerned with the quality of the sperm, the presence or absence of any psychological issues around parenting, and checking the timing of his transits, profections, and solar arcs compared to his partner's chart. Timing in a male chart is not always the key factor. More can, and will go 'wrong' in a female chart, and considering that all we need is sperm from the male, his timing is not going to contradict hers too much. However, occasionally, the male chart is really strong and can outweigh the timing of her chart. This is rare, and usually requires a solid solar arc. I always pay careful attention to the timing of a male chart if he was the one who made the appointment in the first place. It signifies that he takes the lead, and that this question 'when will we get pregnant?' is his and not just hers. In the case of Raylene and Jacques, she made the contact, so her chart is primary, but his had the loudest solar arc, so we pay attention to that. The signatures are different, but men also have an Almuten of Pregnancy, and they have physical or health issues that have an impact on them.

**Jacques' chart**

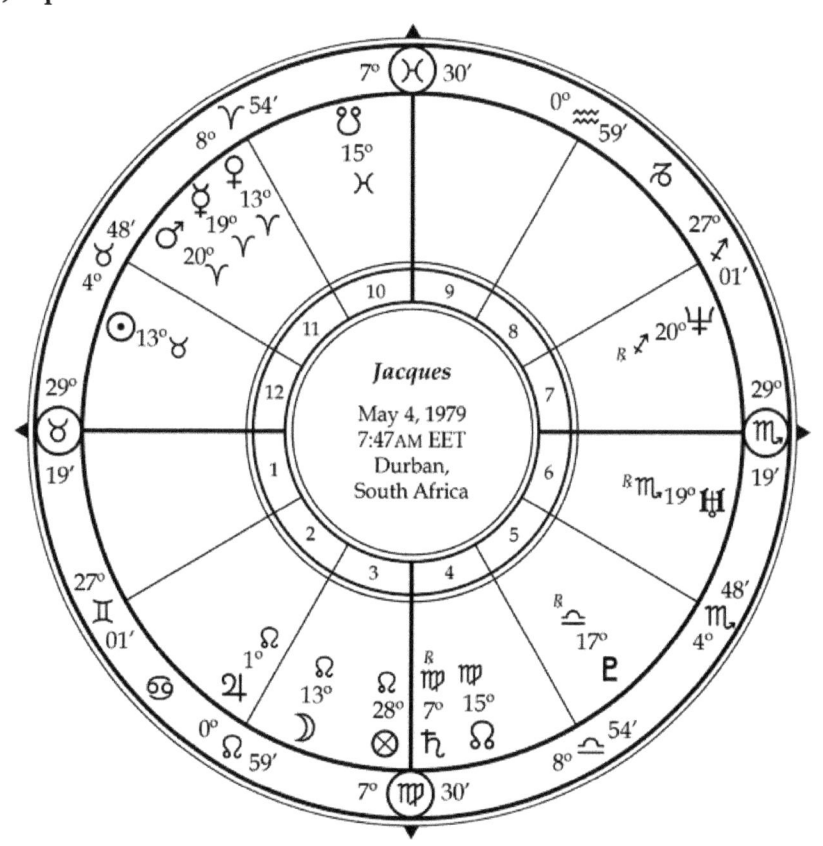

Figure 5.2: Jacques' Chart

86   Fertility Astrology

The first thing to note as a general signature in Jacques' chart (Figure 5.2) is the Sun/Moon/Uranus T-square, with Uranus being in the 6th house (although in the 7th using whole sign houses). The Moon in a man's chart is his physical sperm, his genetic material, the role model for mother and his emotional centre. So one would delineate along the following lines: his Moon is cadent (weak by accidental dignity) in Leo (so no triplicity rulership by essential dignity either). So far this is not promising, but we shouldn't ignore the trine to Venus and the applying conjunction to the Part of Fortune. Jacques does not have the usual signatures for poor sperm health. His Moon is not conjunct Saturn, there is no hard aspect to Mars, and the square to Uranus just means that the fertilisation will take place outside the physical body – either through IVF or that he has a surgical procedure related to his sperm. His Mars is in rulership, which is a good sign, and conjunct Venus and Mercury and all in the 11th house of Good Fortune, which is also the 5th house of his 7th house partner, Raylene. So all looks fairly average with a few problems that are not insurmountable. It was this interpretation that prompted me to be bold with my prediction, even though their client history was unsuccessful and seemingly without hope. The doctor's medical opinion was damning (recommendations for both sperm and egg donation), and the astrology didn't add up to the story that Raylene and Jacques had put before me.

On a psychological level, Jacques' Venus/Pluto speaks of his intimate relationship with Raylene and possible possessive or jealous tendencies, given his highly charged and passionate conjunction of Venus/Mars opposite Pluto in the 5th House. So in consultation with both of them I discussed the need for Raylene to be aware of these feelings and make a concerted effort to create intimacy for them as a couple away from the children, thereby protecting her relationship and the long term happiness of the family. Jacques would feel reassured just knowing that his feelings had been considered. Sometimes this is all it takes for a man to relax about conception.

As it happens, doctors did raise the issue of sperm donation with them, insisting that it was their only chance, and although Jacques really wanted children, he struggled with the idea of another man's contribution, something that harks back to his Venus/Pluto. In 2009 Raylene put pressure on him to consent, and their relationship was put under a huge amount of strain as a result. When I asked Raylene about this particular issue, she said, "He has never said anything about feeling left out due to the children, but his parents got divorced over this very issue. Jacques' father felt the boys' mother spent too much time with them and he was intensely jealous of Jacques' older brother (this is what my mother-in-law has told me). So I know he has 'issues' with this stuff so I put a lot of effort into having 'us' time". To make matters interesting, Jacques also has a Sun/Uranus opposition and a Moon/Uranus square, which means he will need to feel that he still has freedom from the very real and also imagined restrictions that having children brings.

Jacques' Almuten of Pregnancy is co-incidentally also the Sun. His Sun is in Taurus in the 12th house. His triplicity phase rulerships for his major life phases (indicated by Sun in Taurus, an earth sign) are ruled by Venus, Moon, Mars, respectively. He is in the second phase of his life so we look at the Moon. His health, as indicated by his earth Ascendant, also in Taurus, is also ruled by Venus, Moon, Mars, respectively. So the Moon becomes doubly important here.

The Moon in Jacques' chart is in Leo, cadent, square the Sun and Uranus. The Moon also enjoys a trine to his Venus/Mercury/Mars conjunction in the 11th house (derived 5th house of his partner) and a trine to Neptune in his 7th house. Using whole sign house systems, the Moon is also in a wide conjunction with Jupiter by sign, although separating, but applying to a conjunction with the Part of Fortune. So we could say that the second part of his life is going to contain issues to do with his partner's children (Venus/Mercury/Mars in 11th) and with some medical/surgical issues with the square to Uranus in the 6th for his partner also – since Uranus by whole sign is in the 7th. The challenge to the Almuten of Pregnancy is also noted in the square to the Sun, although the aspect is technically separating. It is the separation of the hard aspects and the applying of the conjunction of the Moon to the Part of Fortune that hints at the successful outcome. But before the conjunction to the Part of Fortune, the Moon will first square Uranus, then Mercury, then trine Neptune, to finally square Mars at 20° 57' Aries. It could be anticipated that he might have laparoscopic surgery perhaps (Uranus in 6th) followed by some strife on the homefront (Mercury conjunct Mars) and some sudden unexpected events related to his 7th house partner regarding children.

Also note that a Taurus Ascendant is very physical, given that it is an earth sign, and Taurus is also a very physical sign. So we can expect that Jacques might have physical issues, given his Venus conjunct Mars. The further entanglement with Mercury indicates possible surgery to his vas deferens – the tubes that carry the sperm from the testicle to the seminal sac for ejaculation, functioning in a typical Mercury-type fashion, similar to that of the fallopian tubes in women.

As it happens, in addition to the stresses of the IVF treatments and their home renovations, Jacques underwent surgery to remove three large varicoceles from one of his testicles. The surgery was an initial success, but Jacques had to have it drained again a year later. This swelling or collection of fluid so quickly after the surgery points to the trine to Neptune, as Neptune rules oedemas and lymph drainage functions. Yet, it was also the time of his life when Raylene would fall pregnant.

At the time of the appointment, I noticed that he would be living a profected thirtieth year, and changing to a thirty-first year in the first week of May 2010. His thirtieth year is ruled by Mars, and is a 7th house year, like Raylene's, and thus he is experiencing a year of Venus/Mars/Mercury in opposition to his 5th house Pluto. His Mars is natally in his 11th, so it is a year of his partner's children, and a year of good fortune perhaps. His thirty-first year is an 8th house profection year, ruled by Jupiter, and thus a year of irrevocable change (that is, death and ultimate transformation) and his partner's money. His natal Jupiter is in the 2nd house and sextiles both his Ascendant and his Pluto in the 5th house. So there is a remarkable change in tone from one year to the next, bearing in mind that the changeover happens in the first week of May. By solar arc, on 20 April 2010 he has MC sextile his natal Venus/Jupiter midpoint shortly followed by Venus conjunct his Sun on 27 April 2010 – two very strong signatures, one of which is my personal favourite. Being solar arcs they will be in effect for at least a month, if not two, after that date.

I then looked forty weeks ahead to see if there were signatures that could represent a birth. Flipping ahead to February 2011, I saw that on the 20th Jacques would have his solar arc Sun (his Almuten of Pregnancy) sextile his Moon. By transit Saturn will conjoin his natal 5th house Pluto (a perfect signature for a cesarean birth), and he will also have Uranus conjunct his Ascendant. Both transits speak of the physical risk and trauma of a birth. Uranus is the surgical signature aspecting not only the

Ascendant, but also his 7th house partner, and Saturn plays midwife to a planet in the 5th. Saturn is often referred to by Liz Greene as a midwife, the physical reality that manifests.[81] In male charts I often see the presence of Saturn, either configured on the angles or conjoining the Sun. It seems as though the material burden of raising a child and making them materially secure and safe is placed on males in this way. Also remember that Saturn rules legal documents, including birth certificates and the trust funds and wills that need to be sorted once a child comes into the life of a couple.

**Surprise, Surprise!**
These charts turned out to be an absolute delight. Not only do they contradict conventional medical diagnosis of fertility by resulting in a live birth, they delivered three live births, and were followed by a *second natural pregnancy* that took us all by surprise.

Raylene contacted me soon after the triplets were born, asking for future dates for conception. I thought she was still on the honeymoon high that follows childbirth, when the babies are constantly sleeping and life seems back to normal (i.e. before they are crawling and getting into trouble), but Raylene was eager to complete her family and wanted to try again. At the same time, Jacques enquired about moving to another city and his career, so we picked out more dates, and this time I felt 'performance anxiety' – repeated success with couples whose history is as fraught as theirs makes one very nervous about predicting, especially since they had an expectation of astrology, based on three beautiful little girls.

In January 2012, Raylene sought the advice of a hormone specialist in order to lose the baby weight and to help relieve the symptoms of PCOS that can prevent pregnancy. The result of one of the tests she took revealed a lack of vitamin D, an essential for fertility. This is becoming more common in sunny climates such as South Africa and Australia, where people are concerned about skin cancer, and consequently use sunscreen every day – which prevents the natural production of vitamin D. Raylene started taking vitamin D supplements and had a prescription for a new contraceptive pill to regulate her cycle again, but as she waited for her cycle to begin she noted with dismay that her natural cycle was 120 days – again harking back to her Moon/Neptune opposition and hormonal imbalances. Raylene finally started taking the contraceptive pill on 18

June 2012, and felt very ill as she attended a work conference. In fact, she felt so ill, she returned home early. A throwaway comment from a friend prompted her to take a pregnancy test. It was a decisive positive! Her son was born on 6 February 2013 at 6:17 am in Johannesburg. A fourth child for a couple who were told that they would never be able to conceive with their own eggs and sperm, and without aggressive medical intervention. Let's take a look at the astrology behind this miracle.

First, we go back to see that starting on 20 January 2011 Jacques enjoyed a powerful solar arc North Node conjoining his natal 5th house Pluto. This Pluto can be interpreted as a physical child, the North Node is interpreted by some astrologers as karma (of the positive kind). In May 2012, Jacques had the MC conjunct the 11th house by secondary progression – which I take to indicate a change to the social status of the person in question, and that change contains the content of the 11th house – his partner's house of children. Followed by a long extended window of transits of Jupiter to multiple fertility points in his chart:

> Starting 13 May 2012
> Moon trine the Sun/Jupiter midpoint by secondary progression
> tJupiter sextile the Venus/Jupiter midpoint
> tUranus trine Moon/Jupiter midpoint tJupiter conjunct the ASC
> tJupiter trine Venus/Uranus midpoint
> tJupiter trine natal Jupiter
> tJupiter trine Moon/Uranus midpoint

In May 2012 Jacques would have been thirty-three years old, so his profected ruler for that 10th house year is Jupiter, which is ruled by the Sun (his Almuten of Pregnancy) and sextiles the Ascendant while enjoying a wide conjunction with the Moon. This year was going to be a change of social status (10th house) for him, and it also implies a change of fortune as Jupiter is natally in the 2nd house. As it happens, Raylene confirmed that in that year he received a pay increase as well as a tax rebate of a significant amount. Sometimes it happens that the client receives a pay increase but not a baby, or a baby and not a pay increase. Lucky for Jacques he received both. Their son's due date was 18 February, but he was born on 6 February 2013 at thirty-eight weeks and was a caesarean birth. On 24 February 2013, transiting Jupiter conjoined Jacques' Venus/Jupiter midpoint, and on 26 February 2013 transiting Jupiter sextiled his Moon/Jupiter midpoint.

At first glance, Raylene's transits for the conception of her son were not that strong – no massive solar arcs, no extended line up of transits from Jupiter as in Jacques' chart – but the finish is really strong. Birth and conception both look the same in a chart, and sometimes you get a really strong start and a weak finish, and sometimes it is the other way around. I always advise finding all the strongest times and project forward or backward forty weeks to see if there are correlating signatures. If so, then consider it a fertile bookend. In Raylene's chart, I would have found the strong finish and advised her to try forty weeks before that time, and if not successful to use the strong finish as a start date.

Raylene's conception date was around 26 May 2012. Her transits show the following:

27 April – tJupiter opposes natal Uranus
30 April – tJupiter squares Venus/MC midpoint
20 May – Moon trine Asc by secondary progression
22 May – tPluto trine the Sun (Pluto is a planet in the 5th house natally)

But in June, when she discovered she was pregnant:

6 June – tJupiter trine the Venus/Uranus midpoint
15 June – tJupiter trine natal Jupiter
18 June – tJupiter conjunct Jupiter/Asc midpoint
20 June – tUranus conjunct Venus
20 June – tJupiter trine the Asc

The strong finish for the birth of Raylene's fourth child on 23 February 2013 is shown by her MC making a trine to her Venus/Jupiter midpoint by solar arc.

For the first pregnancy, Jacques' chart had the strongest voice. This is sometimes the case, which is why we always look at both charts. In all types of couples, one chart is often stronger at times, so use these times. The couple are a unit and so what happens in one chart happens to both. In the case of surrogacy clients, I look at all three, but place more focus on the couple raising the child; after all they are the ones who will 'receive' the child. Raylene also had Venus conjunct the Sun by solar arc, but this happened in between the two pregnancies on 13 April 2011. I would have advised her to use this time had she not become pregnant before. I was confident that she would indeed become a mother when she first consulted me, as they both had this signature and not too far apart. The

Venus conjunct the Sun by solar arc is my favourite signature. It is very fertile, and it contains the message that all things dear to the heart – such as love, marriage, babies, and the fulfilment of all things feminine – are being manifested in the solar expression of the person.

**Fixed Stars and Fertility for Raylene and Jacques**
Before we take leave of Raylene and Jacques, I want to review and interpret the most salient and important fixed star indications for this couple to add to what we already know about them in the field of fertility. Raylene has Mirach as her heliacal rising star, which is going to infuse her life with the energy of that star, as the star 'walked the earth' as the Sun rose on the day of her birth. Brady provides the following interpretation of Mirach: 'The themes of this star are receptivity and fertility. If present in your chart it implies that you are open to ideas, willing to be receptive. Some people may mistake this as naivete or innocence, but Mirach is not naive, for she can make use of that which she receives. She is fertile. Her skills are the ability to listen and think and to use this input in a most creative way.'[82] Compounding this, Raylene's Almuten of Pregnancy is the Sun.

Jacques has Hamal as his heliacal rising star. Hamal is not bright enough to be seen rising before the Sun, so it doesn't herald the dawn and thus has a quieter reputation, known as a cosmic star. When Hamal is one's heliacal rising star, Brady interprets it as being able to give one strength of character, independent thought, and motivation.[83] It is interesting that in the first successful pregnancy, it was the solar arc (Venus conjunct his Sun, his Almuten of Pregnancy) in Jacques' chart that manifested – a quiet, strong, supportive, male statement.

On the day Raylene conceived the triplets, the mundane parans indicated Hamal as the heliacal rising star ('Assertiveness, the accident, the unexpected event') and Spica as the heliacal setting star ('An opportunity, a new concept'). Hamal is Jacques's heliacal rising star, and Spica is one of the fertile stars. The stars connected to the Sun, her Almuten of Pregnancy, on this day are the fertile star Acubens ('Issues of the protection or sacredness of life') and, once again, Hamal. Interestingly, the star in paran to the Moon for that period was Ankaa, which indicates 'concern with the wellbeing of families'.[84]

The tonal quality of the stars in parans with a planet shade that planet's transits as well as the quality of the parans in the natal chart. As we saw before with Nancy and Lisa, we will want to take a look at the parans to Jupiter. Jacques has Jupiter in parans with both Spica and Sirius in his natal chart. We would expect that his luck goes beyond the normal limits or expectations, and that he can rely on transits of Jupiter to really push those boundaries. Raylene's natal mundane parans to Jupiter involve Procyon ('finding unexpected solutions') and Ankaa ('success to those who can adapt quickly to new situations'). One could say that Raylene adapted to her situation by trying new solutions to her infertility that other women would consider irrelevant, silly, or naive. Raylene's mundane parans to Jupiter for that period during which she conceived the triplets include contact with Bellatrix ('the unlikely hero'), Alnilam ('crossing over boundaries, bridging the gap between groups'), and Capulus ('success to the aggressive or the cruel'). The parans to Capulus, a very difficult star, is worth noting. After successfully conceiving triplets, Raylene was advised by the very doctors that had said she would not conceive without donor eggs, that she should terminate at least one, preferably two of the embryos to safeguard the pregnancy. This was a cruel and cutting blow for the couple, risking losing all three embryos, for the alleged safety of one of them making it to term. Raylene remained firm, supported by Jacques and his quiet Hamal, and insisted on keeping all three. The quality of the Jupiter that was transiting both their charts during that time carried those themes listed above, and the nature of being both lucky and having to deal with a cruel or difficult decision.

We can compare this to the parans that were linked to Jupiter when Nancy and Lisa were having IVF on the same day. If you remember, Jupiter was the Almuten of Pregnancy for Nancy, and there were no parans for Jupiter on that day using the normal orbs. This is significant, as there was a vacant or muted quality to Jupiter during that transit. However, Mars, Lisa's Almuten of Pregnancy, was in parans with many fertile stars, and Mars was triggering the whole pregnancy by profection and by transit – Jupiter in Lisa's chart, merely supported it.

The Sun is the Almuten of Pregnancy in both Jacques' and Raylene's charts, and so the heliacal rising and setting stars are very important, the mundane parans are equally important, and as transiting Jupiter is always relied on for luck, mercy, and blessings, we would hope that Jupiter has some lovely, fertile parans. Fortunately, for Jacques, his natal Jupiter dictates how transits of Jupiter are going to be received.

When Raylene got pregnant with her fourth child, it was entirely natural, no intervention was needed, and as such no fixed time is recorded for conception. At best, we can use an approximation for the latitude of Johannesburg around the time that Raylene is convinced she conceived. She told me that she is fairly sure of the date 26 May 2012 as this was following a rare occasion of sexual activity, in-between caring for her triplets. Most notable in the mundane heliacal risings and settings during that time period is the attendance of both Algol and Spica. Algol is a notoriously difficult star, symbolised as the head of Medusa, slayed by Perseus as an act of bravery and as part of the foreplay of the seduction of Andromeda:

> ...so hideous were her features, with enormous tusk-like teeth, brazen claws and hissing serpents for hair, that anyone who looked upon them turned to stone. The Gods, who favoured Perseus, provided him with the necessary equipment: Hades gave him a helmet of invisibility, Athena a shield, Hermes winged sandals and a magic wallet in which to carry the head once it have severed from her body... Perseus found the sisters asleep, and not daring to gaze at Medusa, lest she should awaken and petrify him with her glance, he looked at her image reflected in the polished shield, then with a backward stroke of his magic sword he cut off the head and with it started for home.[85]

Algol is also symbolised as the feminine rage of Lilith, first wife of Adam, as Brady reveals:

> In Talmudic law she is the first wife of Adam, Lilith, who left him because she refused to be submissive to his needs. Lilith then fled to paradise and became a demon of the wind. She was considered a curse since she gave sexual pleasure and was the cause of all male wet dreams. This eventually led, in the Jewish, Moslem, and Christian cultures, to the suppression of the sexual woman. Algol thus embodied everything that men feared in the feminine. She is not the mother-face of the goddess but rather the passionate lover or the whore. She is female kundalini energy... Algol in other words, is the wild, raw frightening face of the outraged feminine which has been labelled as demonic or simply evil.[86]

If this star is active in one's natal chart, the brutal nature of life and death are likely ever-present as a background narrative to the life and chart. Yet in Johannesburg, when Raylene was conceiving, the stars that were in parans for that day merely gave the opportunity for participation in those energies in the context of the rulerships of her and Jacques' natal fixed star narratives. Neither of them have Algol prominent in their charts, and so the manifestation is lighter in effect and is more likely to be an outer event, in their environment and not necessarily in their personal lives. It would seem that the presence of Spica as the heliacal setting star, and the fact that the Sun had Dubhe and Rigel in parans suggest that this Algol represented the mating ritual of Perseus, rather than the actual brutality and destruction that comes with this star. Algol is a binary system, which suggests that one could either be represented as the bravery of Perseus and the protection of the Gods or as the head of Medusa slain as her sisters slept.

As an aside, a perusal of the newspapers for that time period did not deliver any particularly destructive event; however, on the topic of feminine rage, a very public debate emerged surrounding a painting of the South African President Jacob Zuma, by Brett Murray, called *The Spear*. It depicts a Lenin-like posture of Zuma, with his genitals exposed, the satire calling to book his many wives, many girlfriends, and his recent rape trial. The story was headline news from 17 May onwards during the time period when her fourth child was conceived and throughout Algol's position as heliacal rising star for the latitude of Johannesburg.

This table shows what the mundane parans looked like in *Starlight* for 26 May 2012 for the heliacal rising and setting stars, the Sun, the Moon, Mercury (representing both the doctor and the astrologer), Venus, and Jupiter (our planet of luck):

Heliacal Rising Star
    Algol – Rising 02 mins 58 secs before sunrise –
    Emotional and destructive times

Heliacal Setting Star
    Spica – Setting 184 mins 27 secs before sunrise –
    An opportunity, a new concept

Sun – The stars in parans with the Sun on this day
   *Setting when Alphard is culminating orb 00 mins 32 secs* –
   Violence, anger, a time of apparent ruthlessness
   *Rising when Fomalhaut is culminating orb 00 mins 37 secs* –
   People and ideals being exalted, or dreams coming undone
   *Setting when Dubhe is rising orb 00 mins 43 secs* –
   The concept of Mother or Father
   *Rising when Rigel is rising orb 01 mins 09 secs* –
   The strength of the government is used to alter, or seek to reform, a situation

Moon – The Emotions of the People
   *Rising when Arcturus is on nadir orb 00 mins 29 secs* –
   Concern for those in need
   *Culminating when Diadem is rising orb 00 mins 47 secs* –
   To care for victims
   *Culminating when Pollux is culminating orb 00 mins 56 secs* –
   Help which is needed fails to arrive
   *Setting when Sirius is setting orb 01 mins 33 secs* –
   A martyr, a person mourned by the common folk

Mercury – Business and the Media
   *Setting when Alderamin is on nadir orb 00 mins 25 secs* –
   Issues of honour and dignity
   *Rising when Algol is rising orb 00 mins 34 secs* –
   Scandal and emotions running high
   *On nadir when Sadalmelek is rising orb 01 mins 40 secs* –
   Over-confidence due to a plan considered to be invincible

Venus – The Social Conventions
   *Setting when Aculeus is rising orb 00 mins 40 secs* –
   Greater social awareness through noticing those in need
   *Culminating when Bellatrix is culminating orb 01 mins 06 secs* –
   Dealing with a rogue
   *On nadir when Bellatrix is On Nadir orb 01 mins 57 secs* –
   Dealing with a rogue

Jupiter – The Type of Action which is Favoured by this Period of Time
*Culminating when Alphecca is on nadir orb 00 mins 09 secs* –
Persistence, with policies or attitude
*Setting when Alcyone is setting orb 00 mins 27 secs* –
Seek the big solution, seek the big picture
*On nadir when Alphecca is culminating orb 00 mins 38 secs* –
Persistence, with policies or attitude
*Setting when Zuben Eschamali is rising orb 01 mins 15 secs* –
The professional politician is successful
*Setting when Acubens is culminating orb 01 mins 28 secs* –
The most creative plan succeeds

One gets the feeling that the fertile stars that attend the Sun, Mercury, Moon, and Jupiter outweigh any negative influence of Algol on that day as nearly all the fertile stars are in attendance to the angles: Alphecca, Acubens, Sadalmelek, Sirius, and Spica. I have included a lot of star detail in this last delineation; I hope that you are becoming more familiar with it and are thus able to assimilate it more easily. It would be a shame to leave out the political back-story that comes through the interpretations of the parans.

**Conclusion**
The addition of the partner's chart can have a significant impact on the ability to predict pregnancy. This exploration of Raylene and Jacques' situation provides one example of how to synthesize the fertile signatures of two individuals seeking to create a family. The next chapter will explore various other cases I've encountered in my practice. The examples will go only so far as to highlight important astrological conditions that may arise as you practise fertility astrology that have not been covered in the longer case studies we have covered so far.

**Notes**
78. Personal email correspondence with Raylene.
79. Ibid.
80. In a follow-up interview with Raylene, I asked her if anything had changed to her home/environment in that year – she said they had substantially renovated their home, and in the process the builders had defaulted and run off with their money and left them with the problem of completing with

new builders. Given that this couple were desperately trying to save all their resources for their ongoing fertility treatment, this seemed like the most unfair blow. At the same time they did a shared donor egg IVF cycle – this did not work out for either party. It is worth noting that the donor would be a 7th house partner (legal partner), and this is reflected in the astrology. All in all, Raylene maintains that the first part of this year was the worst time of her life.

81. Greene, Liz. *Saturn: A New Look at an Old Devil.*
82. *Fixed Stars*, p.54.
83. Ibid p.228.
84. All interpretations in quotes in this paragraph are from *Starlight* software.
85. *Outer Space*, p.227.
86. *Fixed Stars*, p.185

# 6

## Brief Case Studies

In this chapter we'll cover some brief case studies that illuminate some facets of the practice of fertility astrology that you should be aware of as you start to work in this field. I begin with Cindy, a seemingly perfect chart that shows you what everything looks like under ideal circumstances. We then meet Mandy whose chart had an unexpected and extremely fertile signature that resulted in a positive outcome, even if the timing had to be rushed to get there. Then we meet Sue, who presents a case where the prediction does not add up to what actually happens. Finally, Sharon's story shows us how to identify extremely difficult complications in this work. All of these examples provide specific ways of approaching the charts, and reading them together will add to your sense of what it feels like to work in the field of fertility astrology. Let's begin.

**Cindy**
This first case study shows perfect triplicity phase rulership, using methods of directing the luminaries and Ascendant, as per Guido Bonatti's *Liber Astronomiae*, and as per Dorotheus of Sidon's *Carmen Astrologicum*. In this case, a perfect outer planet transit and perfect midpoints resulted in a correct prediction of the day of birth. This prediction was made to an ordinary client, who had come for a general natal consultation, and left with more than she had bargained for!

In Cindy's chart (Figure 6.1), her Almuten of Pregnancy is a wonderful Jupiter in Sagittarius in the 10th house, conjunct the Moon. Her Capricorn Sun in the 11th is lucky and is in the derived 5th house of her partner. She has a diurnal chart so her triplicity phase rulers for her Almuten of Pregnancy are the Sun, Jupiter, Saturn; the Triplicity phase rulers for her Ascendent are Venus, Moon, Mars.

100    Fertility Astrology

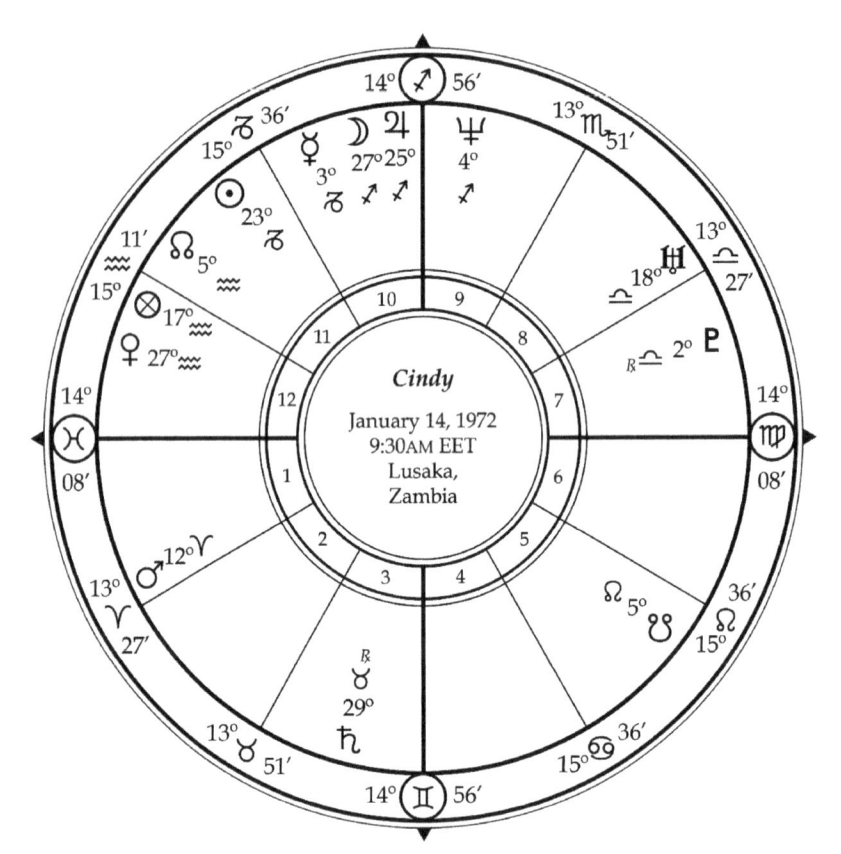

Figure 6.1: Cindy's Chart

By triplicity phase rulership, the Moon and Jupiter rule the time of life when she fell pregnant (January 2003) as the Moon rules second phase of life, beginning at approximately thirty years, and Jupiter rules the second triplicity phase of her Almuten of Pregnancy, which would have changed over at around twenty-six to twenty-seven years of age. That the Moon is conjunct Jupiter in Sagittarius in an angular house indicates very good health during this period, and Jupiter conjunct the Moon indicates wonderful fertility opportunities and good egg production during this phase of her fertility.

The transit of the outer planet Uranus to conjoin her 12th house Venus is punctual and apt given that she was trying to conceive without the tacit agreement or knowledge of her partner (a very common phenomenon). The transit to her Venus/Uranus midpoint is also quite neat and tidy. Her profected year was ruled by Venus in Libra (8th house). So the transit of Uranus to her Venus unlocked the potential of 'irrevocable change' and 'transformation' for that year. Cindy shared that in her previous relationship which lasted some six years, she had not really used conventional/medical contraception, as she was a Catholic, and in spite of sometimes having 'unprotected' sex, she never had a pregnancy scare and had never conceived. She was using the same method of contraception, but this time the astrology lined up.

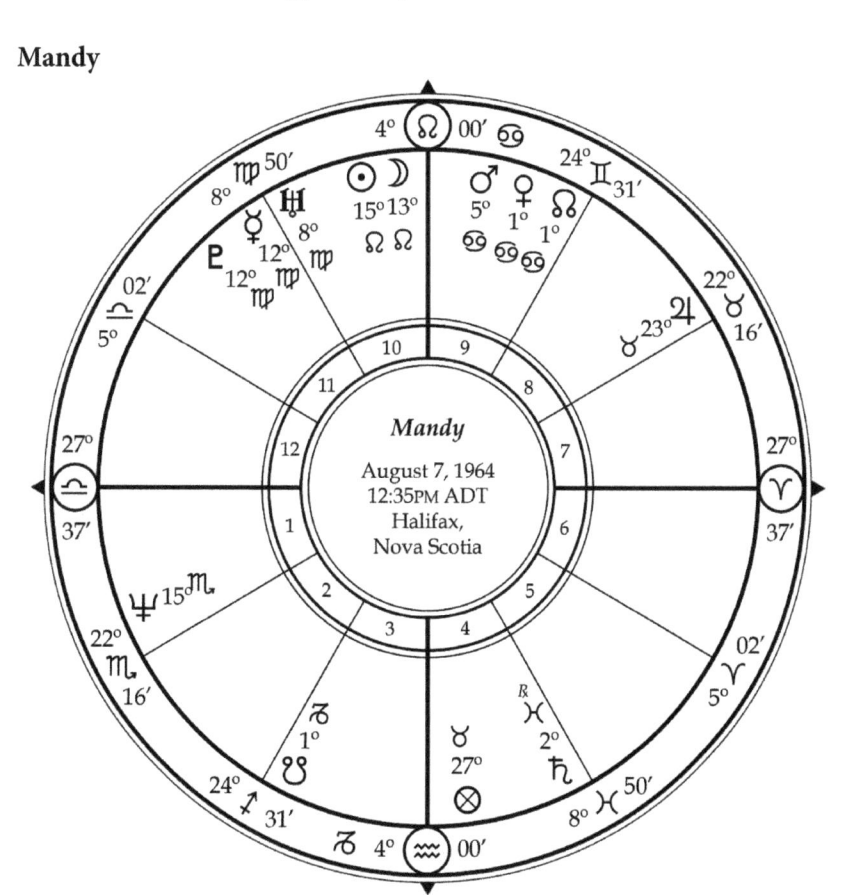

**Mandy**

Figure 6.2: Mandy's Chart

Mandy's chart (Figure 6.2) demonstrates the most obvious fertility signature: a solar arc conjunction of Venus to the Sun. This can only happen once in a lifetime, and it could happen at two years of age or twenty. It just so happened that in Mandy's life, it was happening six weeks after her consultation with me in 2010. Mandy is an educated, intelligent woman, very direct, and no nonsense, but after numerous IVF treatments and using donor eggs, she was at her wit's end. She told me she did not believe at all in astrology and that I was the last resort. And when I told her that the very best time in her whole life was in six weeks time, she almost choked. Financing each round of IVF had crippled this couple, and they had to sacrifice enormously to finance a trip to Cape Town to receive treatment and donor eggs.

What added extra urgency to my interpretation was Mandy's Almuten of Pregnancy: Venus. When an almuten arrives by conjunction to the Sun or Moon in anyone's chart, it is a very strong fertile moment in that person's life. Venus symbolises everything that has to do with feminine wish fulfilment, and in broader terms, social status, love and children. So when Venus is also the almuten, my heart races a little faster. I was extremely confident of my reading and very persuasive in getting her to agree to move heaven and earth for that particular time frame. I had seen this work before, and I was prepared to go out on a limb for this.

Co-incidentally at the time of the cycle, I was also in Cape Town, and I received an urgent phone call from the egg donor company asking me to call Mandy. Things had gone horribly wrong in the donor egg collection, and Mandy was in a terrible state, wanting to fly back home immediately and leave the cycle midway through. I managed to find Mandy and her husband at a restaurant, and we spoke through the astrology again. This time I was more emphatic. The clinic had managed to find her an egg, and all she had to do was commit to having the implantation, but Mandy was really disturbed and wanted to know if she should go ahead and if it would really work. I promised them as a couple that if they did not get pregnant on this cycle, then I would stop practising as an astrologer. I meant it. I thought that if astrology could not come through for me now, when I and my clients needed it to, then I should stop right there and then. I put my faith in my astrology and asked them to do the same. They did. They conceived on that cycle and gave birth to a gorgeous daughter later the next year. I am still practising as an astrologer. This is what Mandy had to say about her experience of astrology and my prediction:

> When I spoke to Nicky about my fertility I really thought it was yet another hopeless undertaking. I had convinced myself, and not without good reason, that my long, unhappy struggle to be a mother

would have a bad ending, and that there was absolutely nothing I could do about it. People say that a definition of insanity is doing the same thing over and over again, whilst expecting a different result. When Nicky told me to sort out a donor egg cycle in six weeks (the normal period of time to arrange a cycle was three to six months) because my horoscope said to do it – well, my take on insanity went one better. I went to South Africa for the fifth time expecting the same result – a negative test or a miscarriage – but I went anyway. There was no hope and no rational reason to go at all – only a resignation that I had to go, even if it was only to say that I had tried everything, honestly everything, and that nothing had worked.

When our carefully chosen and proven egg donor failed so dramatically to produce one egg for our cycle – the agency told me that this had never happened before – I was devastated, but not surprised. And when Nicky and I were able to meet up in Cape Town mid-cycle I managed to be polite to her, but I felt pretty angry, really, even in the face of her obvious concern and her certainty that the eventual outcome would be good. How could a cycle which had started so badly have any prospect of success?

I remember little of what she was saying, other than that she believed it would still work out. So I went ahead with the transfer of two embryos created from anonymous frozen eggs, but I was crying with despair during the procedure. I can tell you that positive thinking is not a necessary requirement of success. When I had my daughter in May 2010, exactly as Nicky had predicted, I was incredulous as well as ecstatic. I don't know how she did it, but I am and will be forever in her debt. My daughter means everything to me. And I say to anyone who asks and who will listen to my story, she would not exist if I had not had a consultation with a fertility astrologer.

The take away here is: the Almuten of Pregnancy conjunct the Sun by solar arc, compounded by Venus being the almuten, amplifying the fertility of this conjunction to the Sun. This was just too good an opportunity to miss. [87]

## Sue

This case study addresses the issue of when the astrology seems to fail – your client does not get pregnant even though you were fairly confident that she would. I searched my database high and low for a chart that 'did not work' so I could demonstrate that sometimes the astrologer isn't always right. I wanted to show an example of where I had made a prediction (with some authority) that did not result in a pregnancy, and I wanted to explore if there was some other astrological angle that I had missed or failed to take into account. I think it is really important to address the failures as well as the success stories, as we can often learn more from them than the successful predictions.

It might be helpful to define 'a successful prediction' in my field. There are two distinct parts to my consultations: one is diagnostic, the other is predicting fertile or lucky times in the future. I usually tell clients that I am around 75 percent correct in the information I give them regarding their fertility, which is different from saying I am 75 percent accurate in my predictions. Astrology can diagnose the physical reasons why the client cannot get pregnant, and if this is the case no amount of timing is going to help. So a correct diagnosis is considered a 'successful' prediction too, even if the outcome is not a live birth. Also, consider that as an astrologer, you are not the medical professional. You rely on the client to give you feedback, and most of the time, people do not call back and tell me if they in fact did get pregnant when I said they would. Sometimes it is just too intimate, and they would rather not acknowledge your participation at all. A lot of the time the partner has no idea the client even went to an astrologer, and the client may wish to deny the active involvement of your skill. Get over the need to be right, get over the need to hear positive feedback; it is not your place to demand it, and it is not your place to write to them or bother them for information regarding their ongoing fertility. This is unethical, and in my opinion, harassment. So my chart base is full of gaps of information that I cannot substantiate either way. Because of my respect for my clients' boundaries, I am working from the data of clients who have been in touch with me of their own accord.

I encountered a number of problems in my search for a chart that didn't work. I have over 3,000 charts, and they can be grouped into categories that look like this:

Aged between twenty–thirty, thirty–forty, and forty–fifty
Issues with fallopian tubes
Issues with implantation
Question about chromosomal quality of eggs
Hormonal (thyroid and other) issues that interfere with normal cycles
Psychological issues – with either person or both
Immune problems – 'killer cell' Sperm issues
Endometriosis and fibroids in the uterus
Uterus abnormalities
Premature ovarian failure, also known as early onset menopause
Secondary infertility (when the client already has one or more children and has struggled to conceive a second or third, etc.)

Some people will present with only one of these issues, some will have multiple factors causing them not to conceive. As you can see, there are enough physical reasons why some people fail to conceive, let alone looking for astrological ones! My client base is made up of people who are struggling to conceive, so it stands to reason that for a lot of them pregnancy is highly unlikely. Making a prediction against these odds is really hard work, and the likelihood of the prediction coming to pass is therefore diminished. The astrologer needs to allow for this. This is not the same as giving up and not making any prediction at all. On the contrary, one needs to get really precise in these cases. The more particular you can be, the more likely the astrology will support your prediction. This is where the diagnostic aspect comes in. The more accurate you are with interpreting the medical conditions, the more your client will get out of the consultation, and they will be able to get the help they need. Then the resulting pregnancy is a reflection of your ability to correctly diagnose, and not simply a matter of timing.

There are many factors that influence whether or not someone will get pregnant. If they have fallopian tubes that are blocked due to a previous STI, and they refuse (on religious or other grounds) to get the proper medical treatment, no amount of predicting the potentially fertile times is going to result in pregnancy. It is a similar situation if they have a recreational drug habit that influences the pituitary gland, as this will influence their likelihood of conceiving. Clients need to take responsibility for their health and lifestyle, and the astrologer needs to

106   Fertility Astrology

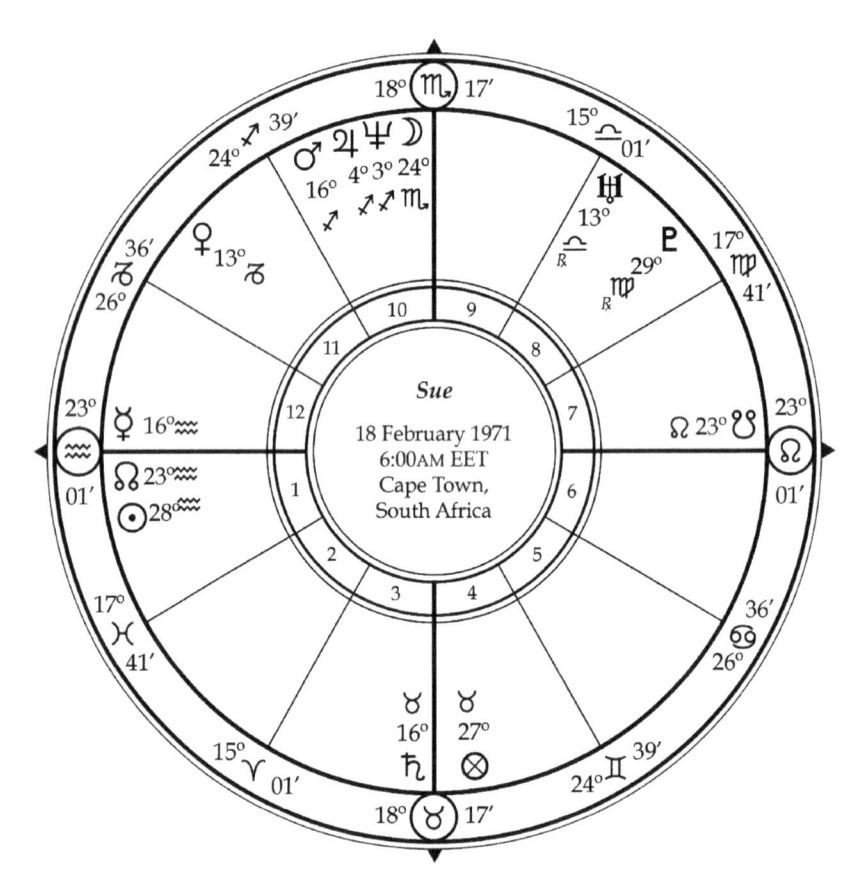

Figure 6.3: Sue's Chart

make a prediction based on how committed and how focused the client actually is. There are too many variables that the astrologer has no control over for them to take the full blame when a prediction does not result in the much-desired pregnancy.

Then there are the cases where the astrology does work, just not in the way you predicted it would! The chart I'd like to share with you is that of Sue (Figure 6.3), who had secondary infertility. Her first child was born prematurely, and she was anxious to complete her family, but she had struggled to have a second pregnancy. After seventeen unsuccessful procedures, Sue found herself at my door. Briefly, her chart reveals Jupiter as the Almuten of Pregnancy, in rulership, angular in the tenth house, and furthermore it forms a sextile with the Ascendent – all looks good so far. The conjunction to Mars might indicate surgery related to becoming pregnant. The conjunction to Neptune hints at something that will not be clear and will undermine her efforts until it is revealed; it also indicates loss, possibly miscarriage. The Moon in Scorpio is a worry, as it is in fall, but the aspect to the Part of Fortune could rescue the situation. The Moon signifies her eggs and her uterus. So one or the other, or both, will be in fall so we can expect some negative anomaly to express itself.

In 2009 when Sue came to see me, I chose the time frame around August/September as a start date for an IVF treatment due to the astrological signatures in her transits. She shared with me that none of her previous IVFs had worked, and, given the conjunction of Neptune to her Almuten of Pregnancy, I noted that there might be something the specialists were missing. Sometimes when medical issues are not clear and headway is not being made, I might suggest to a client that if they have had more than three rounds of unsuccessful treatment at the same clinic, they might consider moving to another medical facility. This is not out of disloyalty to any particular doctor – on the contrary, the relationship between the patient/client and the doctor is sometimes very close, especially from the patient's point of view. The relationship is intimate, so it is difficult to change clinics and get used to another stranger getting personal with your reproductive organs. However, sometimes a change of clinic can mean that your medical record and test results are seen by a new set of eyes, another perspective is gained, and breakthroughs in treatment plans can happen, leading to success where previously only disappointment reigned.

Sue made the change. She went to see a specialist whose expertise is in identifying issues with the uterus in particular. We felt this to be necessary as her chart had the Moon in fall in Scorpio. Her Ascendant – signifying the uterus and the physical body – is Aquarius and Aquarian signatures often present with themes of disassociation, separation, in some cases 'hysteria'. The result of Sue's investigations into the condition of her uterus revealed that she had a septum in her uterus, which meant that each time she had an IVF embryo implantation, the embryo was being placed through her uterus into her body cavity, where conception could not occur.

In the absence of this knowledge, if an astrologer were to examine her chart and make predictions about fortunate times to try treatment, the times would not have worked and would been seen as 'incorrect' from the perspective of the client and the astrologer. This is not a fair comment on astrology. A more correct appraisal would have been that the initial diagnosis of the condition of her uterus, based on the astrological interpretation above, is entirely accurate in the context of what was known at the time.

Sue's story didn't end there. Once the septum to her uterus was repaired, she tried another round of IVF at the time I suggested – around August/September 2009. One of the reasons I was so confident it would work was based on a solar arc of Jupiter (her Almuten of Pregnancy) by sextile to her Venus on 18 May 2010. I took this as a really positive date and subtracted nine months and decided to use the August dates as a start time, since the 'finish' was so powerful. Remember that birth and conception look like the same thing astrologically, and often you will have clients who insist on making use of the next potential time as soon as possible. Under that pressure, I judged that this time frame was the best one we had to work with.

This cycle didn't work. I was confused, and just desperate for her. And yet while working on her chart to find out why it didn't, something miraculous happened. After trying one last round of IVF (that she hadn't told me about), Sue conceived around the middle of October 2009. When she told me in January that she was past her twelve-week scan and that there was a heartbeat and a viable pregnancy, the only thing that concerned me was the solar arc on 18 May 2010. I had a strong feeling that her baby would be born premature, but to introduce this anxiety-loaded issue with her in January would not help the situation. It was too late, and things simply had to work their course. Sue's baby was born prematurely on 18 May 2010, as predicted.

Is this considered an astrological failure? In hindsight obviously not, but to Sue in September 2009, astrology had let her down. Failure is subjective. You can only succeed when you have all the cards in your hands, and the information in front of you.

When I asked Sue what she thought of her consultation with a fertility astrologer, she said she was impressed with the accuracy in terms of what was described about parts of her life and personality that she felt few people knew about her. She felt that this accuracy contributed to her feeling more 'hopeful' and positive about achieving conception and the completion of her family. The words she used to describe how she felt about the advice she was given were: 'those times you pinpointed were like beacons of hope to me; something to work towards, something to plan for'. Sue said she was definitely 'guided' by the astrology, even though she did go for an IVF cycle at a time that wasn't suggested by me.

She said she was impatient, and that even though she wanted it to succeed, deep down in her heart she suspected it wouldn't and as a result she was not as devastated as she had been on previous failed attempts. In total, Sue had five artificial implantations and twelve IVF cycles – seventeen rounds of treatment! Sue now has two children, and in spite of the first cycle with astrology not working, she is a firm supporter of it.

**Sharon**
Sharon's case study provides a detailed look at the profound accuracy of triplicity rulership in terms of life and the medieval concept of the 'Killing Planet' in a chart. Sharon waited seventeen years to become a mother, only to find that shortly after giving birth to a beautiful, lively daughter, she had contracted breast cancer – possibly from the drugs she had taken in her efforts to get pregnant.[86] The health risk factors for fertility treatment are constantly changing, but at the time of writing this book, they include: hyperstimulation of the ovaries; ectopic pregnancies; infection on retrieval or implantation; the unknown impact of estrogen and other drugs, which may cause ovarian or other cancers. Studies about the relationship between IVF and cancer are inconclusive and contradictory at present. The consensus seems to be that it is too soon to make sweeping statements and that a longer period of observation is needed before leaping to conclusions. In addition, women who struggle to conceive also seem to be more likely to develop breast cancer, which should ring alarm bells for astrologers and remind them to look for a Moon/Saturn signature which could be active for those particular women. Note that not all women with Moon/Saturn signatures get breast cancer. Certain psychological and personality traits associated with that signature would indicate a predisposition to negative emotional patterning linked to poor self worth, neglect, issues to do with nurturing, issues to do with relationship to mother, and so on. We always have to assess things very carefully.

110   Fertility Astrology

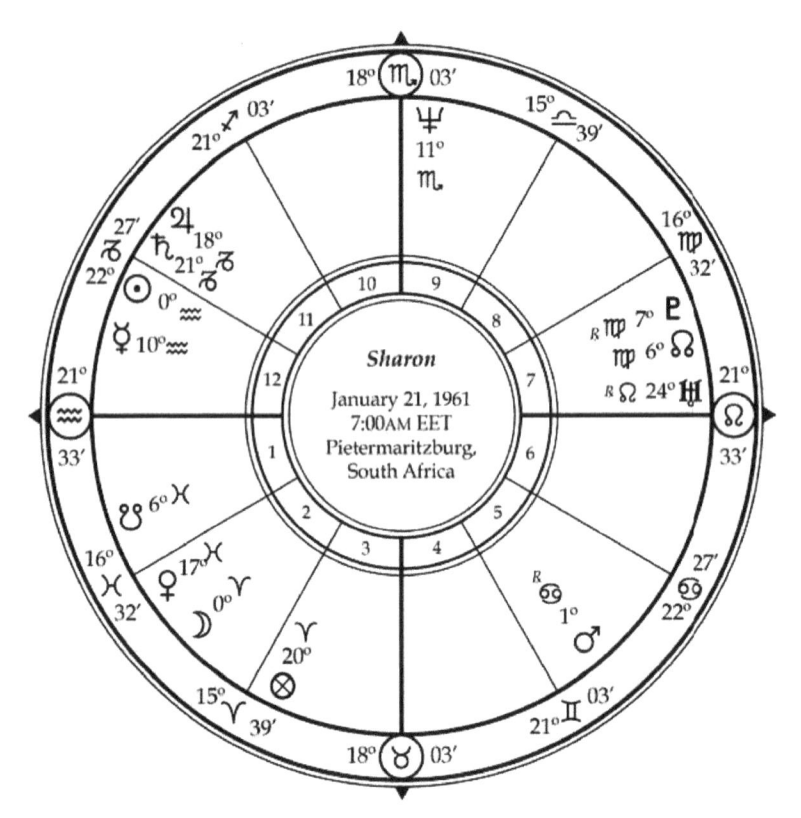

Figure 6.4: Sharon's Chart

The Almuten of Pregnancy in Sharon's chart (Figure 6.4) is Saturn in Capricorn on the cusp of the 12th house. So in her diurnal chart, the triplicity phase rulership of the almuten in an earth sign is going to be: Venus, Moon, Mars. The conditions of each ruler will determine the quality of the ability she has to fall pregnant in these time frames. This triplicity rulership should also take into account the triplicity phase rulership of her life. As we know, significant changes in an individual's circumstances can indicate that a shift into a new triplicity phase has taken place, and we can use those major events to 'mark' the shift in their astrology without having to investigate the Alcocoden and work out the years given in their chart. Sharon's triplicity phase rulership of her life (Aquarius rising, diurnal chart) should take into account Saturn, Mercury, Jupiter, in that order, at the same time as we look at her Almuten of Pregnancy's triplicity phase rulership.

So, her first phase of life looks good, ruled by Saturn in Capricorn, conjunct Jupiter in the 'lucky' 11th house. Health-wise all looks fine, and we can extend this phase until she is in her mid-twenties as a rough guide (using the 'three score and ten rule'). Her Almuten of Pregnancy would rule from fourteen years or onset of menstruation to late twenties, as a rough guide, changing at her Saturn return to the next phase and then again at the age of forty to her final phase of fertility. So there is an overlap in these phases of life and pregnancy that we need to be aware of.

We also need to consider the impact of other almutens on this. For example, a planet can be the almuten of more than one thing in a person's life, depending on how the scoring system evaluates its influence. The Almuten of Profession can sometimes also be the Almuten of Pregnancy, and the Almuten of Pregnancy can also be the 'Killing Planet' in the chart; these issues need to be taken into consideration. In Sharon's chart, however, the Killing Planet is Venus in Pisces, with the triplicity rulers of Venus, Mars, Moon.

Sharon's pregnancy occurred in the last phase of her fertile life – i.e. that triplicity phase of her Almuten of Pregnancy ruled by Mars (in fall in Cancer and consequently in poor condition). Recall that the triplicity phase rulership of her health for that time period (age forty-three) was Mercury, cadent in the 12th in Aquarius, ruled by Saturn, square Neptune in Scorpio. The square to Neptune is going to dictate the quality of life/health for Sharon over the next fifteen years or so, so this needs to be addressed. Neptune is often associated with endocrine issues and imbalances. This could be either natural factors such as a thyroid problem, or self-inflicted as in drug treatment for infertility which radically affects the endocrine system. That this period coincides with a fertile period ruled by Mars in fall indicates not only the hardship in achieving pregnancy and the loss associated with failure, but also that it will not be beneficial to her health.

The story of Sharon's conception is that she tried for seventeen years to become pregnant, used Chlomid and other fertility drugs to stimulate ovulation for numerous artificial inseminations. She finally fell pregnant at the age of forty-two, but had a miscarriage. She fell pregnant again at forty-three and delivered a normal and healthy child in 2003. She then fell pregnant again, but this time the fetus was diagnosed with spinabifida and Down's syndrome and she terminated at five months. Shortly after that traumatic event, Sharon was diagnosed with breast cancer. She had a mastectomy and has been in remission ever since, but has suffered considerable bad health in other areas, such as sinus infections and a bad break of her spine.

The tone of her chart indicated that, although a pregnancy could be achieved, especially on a transit of the Almuten of Pregnancy to a planet in her 5th house, the quality of her life and this fertile phase were not optimal. It also alludes to the possibility that Sharon might have already shifted prematurely into the third and last phase of her life. This could have been brought on by the stillbirth of the second child (albeit a termination, she did go into labour and give birth) and her experience with breast cancer. As a medieval astrologer, this needs to be recognised. The last phase of her life is ruled by Jupiter, in fall, conjunct Saturn. The quality does not improve much, except that she is free of the square of Neptune to the ruler of this phase. Had Sharon been born in the Middle Ages and had she sought the advice of an astrologer, this incident would have had a worse outcome. She would have likely died from breast cancer, if not the stillbirth of the child, and she would have effectively been in the last phase of her life.

Given this, the conjunction of Saturn to Jupiter starts to look interesting. I question whether I should read this as: Sharon gets pregnant in her last fertile phase (Mars in fall), but because of the diagnosis of the breast cancer, do I need to consider that she is in the last triplicity phase of her life? I think I should at least consider it a shift in pace and vitality and suggest that she watches her health very closely.

**Conclusion**

I could share countless more stories here. Hopefully these brief case studies add nuance to the longer studies, giving you more insight into how this practice starts to look when it becomes a typical way for you to interpret charts. In the next chapter, we will review my methods in detail, and in the penultimate chapter, I will provide some specific signatures to aid you as you start to incorporate these methods into your astrological practice.

**Notes**

87. More on this story can be found at www.dailymail.co.uk/femail/article-1348783

# 7

# Methods in Review

In this chapter I revisit in greater detail the techniques I've outlined in previous case studies. Even though the general theory appears here, I highly recommend going back through the case studies carefully to see how I use these theories and techniques in practice. Within this chapter, you will find an initial checklist that covers how to approach a consultation. I then discuss the Almuten of Pregnancy, triplicities, profections, solar arcs, midpoints, fixed stars, and other various astrological techniques and factors that you need to keep in mind to calibrate your fertility consultations with your clients. The chapter that follows this will discuss some prominent astrological signatures to keep in mind.

**Preliminaries**
Before you dive into any astrological techniques, you must first assess the physical and psychological health of your clients, as well as their general lifestyles. Does your client have all the necessary equipment? This seems like an obvious statement, but you would be surprised to hear how often medical investigation reveals missing ovaries, dysfunctional eggs, faulty fallopian tubes, non-existent sperm, etc. First ask the client if they are registered with a clinic or medical doctor, and establish whether or not a semen analysis has been done yet. This is so important – and it is the easiest and most inexpensive test to do – since sperm dysfunction accounts for approximately 20 percent of all fertility issues. Then establish if the fallopian tubes are free from infection and obstruction, and check that your client is ovulating. This is done by testing the blood at regular intervals during her menstrual cycle to see whether she is producing the relevant hormones to trigger ovulation and to sustain pregnancy. Check to see if your client has issues to do with her endocrine system, as conditions such as thyroid problems or diabetes have a direct bearing on her ability to function hormonally.

Then examine any psychological issues that may be involved. Explore your client's feelings about their childhood and what they expect from their own experience of child rearing. Being realistic about limitations and obstacles is helpful in understanding why they want children in the first place, or whether or not they actually have any idea of what it takes to raise a child. Talk about issues such as whether or not the mother will be returning to work and who will take care of the child when she does. Talk about whether or not breastfeeding is going to work or whether the partner will do their share of the night feeds, in which case bottle feeding is probably going to be the source of nourishment. Raise potentially tricky subjects such as what sacrifices each partner is willing to make in order to be available to their partner and the child, and what support they each might need.

Talking about these issues, no matter how far in advance they might seem, actually helps to tease out the real psychological issues that could be inhibiting either partner from fully committing to the process of getting pregnant in the first place. Reassurance that your client is normal, and that fears of 'getting it right' in regard to parenting are fears that each and every parent experiences, can help your client adjust to these new adrenalin rushes that accompany each attempt to get pregnant.

Talk to your client about the temporary loss of a sexual relationship and what that might mean in their romantic relationship. What are her and her partner's expectations? It is normal for most couples to go through stages of sexual disinterest during the pregnancy, due to tiredness, morning/evening sickness, loss of self-esteem due to changes in body shape, loss of libido due to psychological disturbances (for men this is often because of the merging image of mother and seductress). It is also normal to continue to have a vigorous and healthy sexual relationship until hours before, and sometimes even during, the delivery. There is no prescription and each couple is different.

Most couples complain about a loss of sexual activity in the first two years after a child is born. Usually this is to do with low energy levels, as children are naturally demanding and totally time consuming. Time for romance seems like an impossibility. Also, physical discomfort during sexual intercourse is sometimes experienced, especially if the woman has had stitches or an episiotomy. Sometimes it takes longer to heal than the prescribed six weeks, and partners need to be aware that the fear associated with experiencing pain in that sensitive area can cause all sorts of sexual dysfunction. Couples need to be aware of the importance of good communication in order to deal with this potentially sensitive issue with maturity and understanding. A woman often loses her entire sexual identity in the process of giving birth and needs time to collect herself again in this regard. Re-discovering sexuality after birth can be deeply bonding for the new parents, and it contributes greatly to the bonding experience of mother-father-child if this can be brokered without fallout.

Then it is time to ask about your client's domestic situation, as it so often has a huge impact on the ability to get pregnant. Explore the nature of the primary relationship that your client is engaged in, and see if there is any imbalance of power that needs to be addressed. Now is the time to sort these issues out. They could be impeding the conception in the first place! Financial insecurity is one of the major factors of infertility in my research, so pay attention to the needs of both partners in this relationship – *secure the nest!*

Next, *fence the nest!* Pay attention to the other secondary family relationships and their dynamics. Are there any issues to be resolved in the internal and external family dynamic, such as an overbearing mother-in-law or interfering aunt/sister? Talking about these family members in such a light will tease out any unresolved feuds and vendettas that will definitely cause everybody a good deal of stress once the baby comes. It is best if the couple are fully aware that a baby also has a right to establish relationships with members of the whole family, not just mum and dad.

These topics may go without saying, or seem like an odd place to start a consultation, yet they are important preliminaries to discuss as you need to know what you are working with before you can apply the astrology. Once you are ready to do that, the following checklist can help guide you through the various techniques discussed in the case studies.

## Checklist of astrological considerations

### Almuten of Pregnancy

- Examine the condition of the Almuten of Pregnancy. An Almuten in good condition is typically: angular, in rulership, has good aspects, in the 5th house, or a combination thereof.

- Check if the Almuten of Pregnancy has good or fertile stars in parans.

**Triplicity Ruler of Ascendant and Luminary**
- Is the condition, or dignity, of the triplicity ruler of this particular phase of life supportive of your client wanting to get pregnant?
- Is her health (Ascendant) going to bring issues to bear, or are the general events in her life (main luminary) going to have an impact in some way?
- Is the triplicity ruler of her Almuten of Pregnancy going to be supportive or work against her? Consider the condition and make a judgement.

**Profected year**
- Is the ruler of the profected year the Almuten of Pregnancy? If not, does the ruler aspect the Almuten?
- Is it a 1st, 7th, 5th, or 11th house year?
- Does the profected house contain the Almuten of Pregnancy?

**Solar Arcs**
- Are benefics aspecting the 1st, 7th, 5th, or 11th houses?
- Are benefics aspecting the Sun? The Moon?
- Are benefics aspecting Almuten of Pregnancy or one another?
- Are benefics aspecting fertile midpoints?

**Solar Return**
- Is the profected house ruler well aspected and placed in the solar return chart, i.e., aspecting the Almuten of Pregnancy, aspecting the Ascendant or the 1st, 5th, or 11th house cusp?
- Is the ruler of the solar return in the 1st, 5th, or 11th house?
- Is the 5th house free or besieged?

**Transits**
- Which house is the Almuten of Pregnancy aspecting by transit?
- Does the Almuten of Pregnancy aspect by transit the 1st, 5th, or 11th house?

- Is the Almuten of Pregnancy receiving current aspects from other transiting planets that reduce its effectiveness or strength?
- Does the transiting planet that you are investigating trigger any profected ruler or a house that contains the Almuten of Pregnancy?

**Midpoints**
- Are any significant midpoints activated?

**Fixed stars**
- Are any fertile fixed stars making significant contact to your clients' charts during the fertile time periods already highlighted using the methods above?
- Check the mundane parans for fertile stars.

**Firdaria**
- This technique, although not discussed in the case studies, is used by advanced medieval astrologers. Does the firdaria, sub- or main period, contain the Almuten of Pregnancy, or are any of the houses ruled by the main or sub-period linked to the 5th or 11th house?

Now that we have covered the essential checklist, let's revisit these areas in more detail.

**Reason for using the Almuten of Pregnancy**
Sometimes it is hard to interpret how likely someone is to fall pregnant just by a glance at the chart. Most modern astrologers would simply look to the ruler of the 5th house to assess the possibility of achieving a conception. Others might go to the Ascendant to see if the body is healthy enough. Others might look to the Moon and her aspects, in particular to Jupiter or Venus. But what if the Moon trines Jupiter in a natal chart, yet the 5th house is ruled by Saturn or has Saturn present in the house? How do you decide which is more important or relevant? Is Saturn always a bad planet? Does a transit of Saturn to the 5th house mean that a pregnancy is not possible?[88]

Thankfully, there is a technique from Persian astrologer Omar of Tiberias, to assist us in making a judgement on the likelihood of pregnancy in a natal chart.[89] Omar and other Arabic–era astrologers were fond of using something called an almuten, also known as *Mubtazz* (loose translation, 'victor'), meaning, the planet that has the most dignity over the matter at hand. You construct a table of points in the chart related to a certain facet of life, and then add up the essential dignities of all the planets at all those selected points and the 'winner', the one with the greatest amount of dignity, is the almuten. Omar of Tiberias calculates the Almuten of Pregnancy as follows:

> For pregnancy look at the Ascendant and its lord, and the Moon and the lord of her house, also the fifth and its lord, and whatever planets may be in the fifth house, and Jupiter. Also, one examines the Almuten over these places; and one introduces into this signification, the eleventh house and the place of Venus. Therefore, when you are asked concerning pregnancy, whether there may be one or not, look at the Almuten over the Ascendant and the Almuten over these places, whether there may be a conjunction, translation, or collection between them according to the fourteen suitable combinations, and this [combination] should be with the soundness of the receiving planet and the received planet; this signifies that there will be a pregnancy here.[90]

So we can gather from Omar of Tiberias that the idea is to interpret aspects of the almuten in the traditional rulership fashion of mutual reception taking dignity, accidental or otherwise, into account. Based on Omar of Tiberias, the points I use in my particular Almuten of Pregnancy are:

Degree of the Asc
Ruler of the Asc
Degree of the Moon
Ruler of the Moon
Degree of Jupiter
Degree of 5th house
Ruler of 5th house
Degree of any planet in the 5th house

Add up the dignities using five points for rulership, four for exaltation, three for all three triplicities, two for term and one point for face. It is relatively easy to program Solar Fire to do this, so I encourage you to take the time to do it, and use it in your practice.

It can happen that either Saturn or Mars become the Almuten of Pregnancy. When this occurs it is more fortunate that you may imagine, as it reduces the number of malefics that interfere with pregnancy by half. If the almuten is Mars, a transit of Mars to the 5th house becomes a desired transit, not something to be feared, nor an obstacle to fertility. Same thing for Saturn.

In predictive work, profected houses, and solar return rulerships suddenly take on a new complexion. Mars becomes something positive, Saturn is welcomed to the Ascendant.

If the almuten is Saturn and is aspected by Jupiter, Venus, or the Part of Fortune, then you would predict a high possibility that the native will achieve pregnancy in due course. The almuten works for both male and female charts. Likewise if you see that the almuten (Saturn for example) is conjunct Mars, then we would tone down the expectation that pregnancy is going to happen in an easy and normal fashion.

**Triplicity**
This is not intended to be a definitive comment on the history of medieval techniques, nor a comprehensive commentary on the way in which authors such as Vettius Valens and Dorotheus of Sidon handled the idea of trigon lords or triplicity phase rulers, but a short statement might be helpful.

I practise a version of astrology which mostly uses medieval techniques from a range of authors. I favour Guido Bonatti, Dorotheus of Sidon, Omar of Tiberias, to name just a few. One of things I especially love about medieval astrology is its sense of destiny and its ability to predict. One of the central tenets of medieval astrology is that you cannot predict what is not in the chart, so if someone is not born to be king, they will not become king. Really simple thinking. Similarly, the length of life is given in the chart and all things are predicted from that.

The astrology of Vettius Valens, writing in the middle of the second century CE, leans toward fatedness, a kind of Stoicism, as does (to some extent) that of Dorotheus of Sidon. Like other Stoics of the time, Valens, believed that you had 'choice' or free will, until you chose – then you had to live with the consequence of that choice. Dorotheus demonstrates that he believed that the chart contained a certain destiny, but his inclusion of a chapter on katarchic astrology, which deals with electional charts for successful outcomes, also shows that he thought it benefitted the person to know what lay ahead, so that they might accept their fate more readily and work with the chart and its destiny, rather than trying to fight it.

Dorotheus based his ideas on trigon lords (triplicity rulers of the Ascendant, luminaries, etc.) on an older system of two trigon lords. Most of his predictive work demonstrates an adherence to this system of using two trigon lords, and not three. However, in a text translated from Arabic, there appears to be a contradiction:

> If the first of the lords of Venus's triplicity is in a good place and the second in a bad place, then this condition in the matter of women is good in the beginning of his age, and in the last it is bad, because the first of the lords of Venus's triplicity indicates the first years, the second indicates the middle years and the third indicates the end of life.[91]

By the time Bonatti takes up the idea of triplicity phase rulership, all three triplicity rulers for three phases of life are used.

Now that medical science has altered possible life expectancies, we actually do need to readdress the issue of calculating the length of life from the chart. These advances have led us to regard the astrological length of life as more of an indicator of vitality and physical energy than a literal length of life. Charts respond to this shift and punctual changes in the pace of life in natal charts have been researched and recorded. A good example of this is the chart of Nelson Mandela, the late former President of South Africa, who was given some eighty-five astrological years. Although he did not physically die at age eighty-five, he announced his official retirement from public life at that time.

In my own practice, I started looking at Bonatti's idea of using the Ascendant to direct the three phases of life by triplicity, as physical health is important to medical matters, in particular fertility. Bonatti practised in the Middle Ages in Italy, and he would have been very familiar with the idea that your physical location and local environment have a profound effect on your physical health – just think of the plagues and the filth in the streets of medieval Rome, and you will begin to understand that link more clearly.

Ptolemy favoured directing the main luminary (Sun in diurnal charts, Moon in nocturnal charts), which is also applicable. The ability to which we are able to express our solar self in the world can have an effect on personal circumstance, such as wealth and station, which favours better conditions for fertility and health in general. I think this is a social expression, and I find it does have an impact on couples and how they feel about becoming parents. Most clients appreciate that it takes money and time to raise a child and that if you have access to neither, then it is not going to be easy. I am not saying one needs to be rich to conceive, but access to resources makes it easier – easier to conceive in the first place and better medical care later on in the process.

Another example of the need to revise medieval ideas for modern contexts is a well-documented signature: that those born with Moon (main luminary) conjunct Saturn will have a hard time in life due to the mother most likely being a slave, and therefore the conditions of birth and youth are detrimental, and the prospects limited because of the station of life into which one was born.[92] The concept of slavery is outmoded, but we see remnants of it in things like 'wage slavery' or people who are forced to work multiple jobs to make ends meet. Sometimes people can even be wealthy with this signature, but they express it in terms of fears related to not having enough resources (time, money, or love). Again, this is another instance where we need to update medieval astrology into something that incorporates modern expressions of being in the twenty-first century.

In terms of directing by triplicity for fertility work, I find that I favour the Ascendant, as it is in a physical body that a pregnancy must happen, and in first world countries most people have access to health and social programs that offer them medical care to conceive as part of a human rights charter. For example, it is entrenched in the charter (in EU and UK) that all citizens have the right to have a child, and so the government has to support the right to try and conceive, which means that a native with the previously mentioned Moon/Saturn would fare much better now than they would have done in the Middle Ages.

There is a phenomenon called 'secondary infertility', which is when a couple successfully get pregnant without any assistance or intervention and deliver a live birth with no trouble at all, and then struggle to achieve a second pregnancy. I have often wondered about this, as the physical circumstances are often the same, the mother is a similar age (usually three years after the first) and the father is usually in similar health, the financial situation or lifestyle is usually improving, and yet these couples are not conceiving. Astrology tells us that we do not experience our whole chart at once, nor do we experience everything contained in it on a daily or annual basis. So, how do we decide when some signatures play a larger or smaller role in a particular phase of life? And is it possible for someone to be both fertile and infertile?

Directing the chart by triplicity shows that there are areas of life that also go through phases. So, if the astrologer was looking at the part of wealth, they might find that one can be born rich, then lose it all, only to regain some in the last phase of life. Or, one can be born rich, lose it all in the middle years and lose even more in the last phase. Or, be born poor, stay poor in the middle years and become rich in the last phase of life. If the natal chart doesn't contain the signature that indicates winning the lotto, then sadly it won't come to pass.

The chart can only express what is contained in it. But what we learn from this is that things are not static, situations can change regarding health, wealth, and relationships and astrologers have devised a way to interpret this by directing points in the chart (luminaries, Ascendant, almutens, and so on).

After thinking deeply about the issue of secondary infertility, I decided that there must be an astrological reason for the change in the fertility status of an individual, and that it may just be that there are three fertility phases also that apply to a person's life and chart. So I decided to calculate the Almuten of Pregnancy (which is conceptually similar to an Arabic Part or Lot) and direct it according to its triplicity phase rulers. I also determined that a woman's fertile life is from age twelve to fifty (roughly) and so the first phase is from age twelve to twenty-six or twenty-seven, the second phase from age twenty-six or twenty-seven to thirty-eight, and the last phase from age thirty-eight to fifty years. I would look at the triplicity rulers of the almuten, according to the system of the three Dorothean triplicities, ordered appropriately according to sect (see p.31 for Table of Dorothean Triplicities), and use them to describe the nature of these phases. The dignity of that particular planet in the natal chart would enable me to make accurate statements about the quality of each phase of a woman's fertile years.

This technique shows that fertility is not static; it can change even if someone's health is good and remains the same. I have seen many clients who have sudden, unexpected pregnancies in the first phase of life, and then struggle to achieve pregnancy with the same partner in the second. Ironically, some women then fall pregnant in the third phase, around menopause, when the hormonal functioning suddenly starts changing.

It is not a definitive timing technique, as each woman has her own fertility time clock based on her own unique ovarian reserve. Even so, it is a powerful indicator of the timeframe in which the woman is more likely to achieve pregnancy. This helps when you are talking to younger women, usually about love and career matters, and you notice that their fertile years are in the first phase of life; it might be beneficial for them to know that and not put off motherhood until later in life – if being a mother is a 'deal breaker'.

Sometimes, as an astrologer, you have to listen to the stories of their journey to decide for yourself if they have changed fertility or life phase. Recall Sharon, in the previous chapter, who tried for seventeen years to get pregnant without success, then suddenly and quite naturally found herself pregnant twice at the ages of forty-five and forty-six. When paying more attention to the triplicity phase rulership of her Ascendant and her main luminary, it was apparent that she was in the last phase of her life, which coincided with the last triplicity phase rulership of her fertile life. She developed breast cancer shortly after the second pregnancy was terminated, and had a mastectomy while trying to keep up with her toddler. Her case reminds astrologers that a change in triplicity phase rulership describes a change in the tone or the quality of the life of the native, and a change in the triplicity ruler of the Almuten of Pregnancy likewise describes a change in the fertile potential in the chart.

**Annual Profections – Lord of the Year**
Our charts are not expressed in their totality each and every day of each and every year. Traditional astrologers used the timing technique called profections as a means to rank the power of the year's transits to determine which ones would result in events for a given native. It is a simple and effective tool to use to fine-tune your predictions.

The method of employing profections can be quite easy once you get used to it. First and foremost, you must always use whole sign houses to calculate the profection year ruler. This is a non-negotiable facet of this technique, and failure to adhere to this rule will result in faulty predictions.

Second, understand that each solar year of your client's life corresponds to a sign in the natal chart. The sign in which the Ascendant falls forms the beginning of the profection calculation. From the Ascendant count one sign/house for each year of your client's age. So the Ascendant to the 2nd house is their first year, from the 2nd house to the 3rd house is their second year and so on, going around the chart for each year of your client's current age. For example, when a client is twelve years old (having gone completely around the chart) they will be living a 1st house year again, and at forty-five they will live a 10th house year.

Then, note the traditional planetary ruler of the sign on the cusp of that house represented by the profection year. This planet becomes the 'profection year ruler' and is 'turned on', so to speak. Then note which house the ruler occupies natally and what aspects the ruler has to other planets in the natal chart. These houses and aspects form the focus for the year ahead and inform you of the quality of the year. Solar arcs and transits (especially those involving the profection year ruler or the sign of the profection house) will then form a tighter timing mechanism where you can narrow down when in that particular year events are likely to occur. A more detailed description of natal profections can be found in Ben Dykes' book *Introduction to Traditional Astrology: Abu Ma'shar and al-Qabisi*.[93]

**Midpoints**

Reinhold Ebertin's book *The Combination of Stellar Influences* is one of the best resources for medical or health astrology.[94] Its directory format makes it easy to use, and the research and observations – regarding topics such as birth, motherhood, hormonal issues, endocrine malfunctioning, ovulation, and formation of sperm – are detailed without being prescriptive, and general without being vague. I highly recommend *COSI* in fertility astrology to help understand the nuances of issues at any given stage of the treatment of infertility. Planets can trigger particular midpoints by solar arc, transit or progression, and these midpoints are sensitive and reliable indicators. It has been shown in my research that the Almuten of Pregnancy, or transiting planet, is frequently found to be actively triggering one or more of these midpoints by transit, solar arc, or progression. In my fertility work, the most reliable and consistent midpoint is Venus/Uranus, in the context of the fertility myth of Uranus and the disembodied/disassociated nonsexual reproduction that accompanies medical and technological treatment. This is a highly sensitive midpoint that also responds to a transit of Saturn. In this context Saturn behaves as a spiritual midwife, manifests the pregnancy and prevents it from being swallowed by Uranus. So any solar arc or transit will highlight a potentially fertile time. The following midpoints come up regularly in transit or secondary/tertiary progressions:

| | |
|---|---|
| Venus/Moon | Almuten of Pregnancy/Moon |
| Venus/Sun | Jupiter/Sun |
| Venus/ASC | Jupiter/Moon |
| Venus/MC | Jupiter/ASC |
| Venus/Jupiter | Jupiter/MC |
| Venus/Mars | Uranus/Moon |
| Almuten of Pregnancy/Venus | Mars/Saturn |
| Almuten of Pregnancy/Jupiter | Saturn/Uranus |

**Fixed Stars**

From Platonic cosmology, we receive an image of the path of the incarnating soul. Originating in the realm of the fixed stars, the soul slowly descends through the spheres of the planets until the Moon deposits them on earth during a full or new Moon. A traditional astrology that does not take into account the fixed stars is incomplete. We learn from the creation myth in Plato's *Timaeus* that earth functions as a 'receptacle' (or 'chora') and that this receptive womb-like space is constantly in flux, with the elements of air, fire, earth, and water being in unequal parts at all times and not static. The Demiurge and Daimons can give you a life (natal chart), but when and where you arrive on earth will determine your interaction (depicted through your chart) with the elemental environment in which you find yourself.

For Gregory Shaw, this *receptacle* need not be merely space and location; he suggests an active participation and it is his understanding that the chora behaves like a 'nurse' (*tithene*) of all generations, and in turn helps us understand the conditions that existed before the formation of the elements (air, water, fire, earth) as we understand them to be.[95]

Taking these scholarly comments to their logical conclusion, using the entire sky in astrology will help us understand the nature of our 'chora' and can show us how we can be supported by the narratives that were active at the location of our birth.

Fixed stars are all about location. They are extremely sensitive to the latitude, and they are also particularly visual. The whole night sky forms the stage on which the planets move, providing the backdrop to the unfolding drama. Planets can only move within the belt of the ecliptic – the disc plane of our solar system – thus dividing the sky into a hierarchy of place and space. Some stars near the poles are never animated by the planets, and some constellations are constantly being cast in leading roles. People often assume fixed stars are located at specific degrees of the ecliptic. This is an error stemming from Ptolemy's projection of stars onto the ecliptic, which distorts the visual relationships between the fixed star points and the planetary narratives – and, in fact, this was actually never intended to be astrological, but a manoeuvre to help him measure parallax!

Only fifteen stars, known as the Behenian fixed stars, are close enough to the ecliptic to factor into this perspective of fixed star work. The rest of the sky will never come close to that narrow path of the Sun, which leaves out so many sky stories from predictive work. The paran methodology, as recaptured by Bernadette Brady, allows for a multi-dimensional experience of stars to finally rejoin our interpretive tool kit. Parans allow the horizon to become dynamic, and are inclusive of these stars and constellations that will never 'literally' cross the ecliptic. In the effort to provide efficient, precise, and predictive answers for my clients, I incorporate the fixed stars into my consultations.

Finally, you will find that some clients present you with some interesting choices in their treatment. For example, in my experience, American clients do not seem averse to travelling long distances, to other cities and countries, in order to receive the treatment they need. On the whole, these clients do their research and find doctors from around the world who specialise in treating the specific type of infertility that they suffer from. When this opportunity presents itself, it is helpful to use fixed stars to see what location is more fertile at that time. I would look to the heliacal rising stars and those on the angles of the week/days when implantation is most probable, and then I would look at the parans to the

Almuten of Pregnancy and those of Mercury. I would judge the better location and be able to help the client make up their mind as to where to have the cycle done, as well as when.

As you become more adept at using both traditional astrology in combination with sidereal or fixed star astrology, you will introduce the option of choosing the location of treatment (latitude) in order to maximise the timing of the planetary transits for timing.

- If the heliacal rising star is favourable for conception, then it bodes well, since heliacal rising stars are powerful in their ability to describe the type of energy active at that location at that time. This is similar to the concept of chart rulership.

- If the Almuten of Pregnancy has fertile stars in parans, but the heliacal rising star is definitely not a fertile one, then one should be cautious about the likelihood of a successful conception, especially since most of the time fertility astrology serves clients who are challenged in this regard. This is not to say that it cannot happen, because the stars work in co-operation with each other, and this might outweigh the heliacal rising, but it is not common.

- If the Almuten has no stars in parans (according to the default setting of 2 minutes of orb) then you should be wary. Recall the chapter with Nancy and Lisa: in Nancy's unsuccessful IVF, her Almuten of Pregnancy had no stars in parans on that day; there were no fertile sky representatives to intercede on her behalf, so her attempt was unheeded by the gods, and her desire was thwarted.

- Assessing the parans to Mercury is also important. Mercury is the signifier for the doctor, the fallopian tubes, and the astrologer. He will go between the worlds to the other place, where mortals are not allowed, to return with an incoming soul. So, parans to Mercury are extremely important. If, for example, Mercury has parans with lucky stars, such as Sadalmelek and Sadalsuud, then it would seem that this doctor, these tubes, and this astrologer are all lucky and 'favoured by the King' according to the myths that accompany these particular stars.

To cite a specific example in context, consider Cape Town at the latitude of 33 degrees south. The fertile pair of stars, Sadalmelek and Sadalsuud, become the heliacal rising stars in Cape Town each year punctually between February 15 and 25. According to local birth statistics, the highest peak in live births happens at the end of September! This is a strong reminder of the fertile potential that these stars bring to that latitude. We can conclude therefore that at that time of year, Cape Town is a fertile place.

## Conclusion

Each of these methods provides a particular strength to the prediction of pregnancy. Perhaps you have already been using one or more of them. Hopefully you can now see the theoretical foundations for my practice and begin to incorporate them into your own work. When I first began writing this book, I wanted my text to be free from the genre of cookbook astrology because as you have seen until now, each client presents you with unique situations that cannot be flattened out with generic signatures. However, as writing progressed, I found that it would actually be useful to provide a sense of what some signatures mean, with the caveat that you will need to synthesize them and modify them as your own proficiency improves. So with that in mind, let's turn to some common astrological signatures you will find in fertility consultations.

### Notes
88. An example of this is in the charts of Amanda (Chapter Four) and Sharon (Chapter Seven), where the Almuten of Pregnancy is a malefic and a transit or profection triggers a positive outcome. Another astrologer might have been reluctant to be so positive, not knowing that Saturn was welcome in the 5th house by transit, especially in Sharon's chart.
89. *Three Books on Nativities*, p.90.
90. Ibid.
91. *Carmen Astrologium*, 2.3.21, p.200.
92. See the *Liber Hermetis*.
93. Dykes, B. *Introduction to Traditional Astrology: Abu Ma'shar and al-Qabisi*.
94. *COSI*.
95. Shaw, Gregory. 'The Chora of the Timaeus and Iamblichean Theurgy.' (*Horizons*, 2012: p.110).

# 8

## Signatures of Fertility

These signatures are a result of my personal, embodied experience of infertility and the medical treatment thereof (including artificial insemination, drug treatment to stimulate ovulation, laparoscopies, and cycles of IVF), and my conscious observation of the symbolism throughout my astrological counselling experience. Further research of a few thousand charts has also informed my practice and my understanding of how the symbolism works in the field of fertility. It is important to bear in mind when talking about fertile signatures in charts, that we are not delineating each and every meaning behind a signature, but only those factors which have an impact on fertility as shown in the results of my research.

Astrological symbolism can manifest in varying degrees and in different ways. The narrative might be the same (think crime story), but the role that the client plays might be different (think victim or murderer). Astrological narratives, then, allow for other people to fulfil certain signatures in the chart; the client does not personally manifest all the signatures in their own personal stories or medical health history – which gives credence to the idea that having many social relationships in your life leads to good health, especially if some of your friends and family (and even pets) manifest some of your signatures for your vicarious experience!

Some signatures are extremely literal in their manifestation. However, as all practising astrologers will know, sometimes the symbolism is literal, sometimes it has a deeper resonance. For example, a transit of Saturn on the Ascendant could mean a visit to the dentist, but sometimes it signifies the inner awareness of the need to isolate oneself from others, or to feel the burden of the responsibility of a 7th house partner. Our clients sometimes experience both the literal visit to the dentist and the isolation from a peer group simultaneously.

Some clients will only experience the literal meanings, and never develop the awareness to dig a little deeper; it is our job to help them do so. In my opinion, this is where we find the spiritual aspect of astrology; in the action of taking the interpretation of the literal to the realm of the symbolic, and in turning the client to see things from another perspective so that they are able to see the need to change, the need to individuate, and to take responsibility for their own charts and lives. It is incumbent upon each astrologer to take the interpretation of the symbolism to the classroom of 'what now?' It is not enough to leave the client with the interpretation of their Moon/Saturn aspect as 'a narrative of not enough'. We need to unpack what that means to them and show them how to approach this narrative with hope and confidence, and return this process to the literal interpretation of moral action required in order to overcome or deal with these difficult narratives. Before entering into specific signatures, then, it is useful to review an example of how the fourfold hermeneutic works in astrological symbolism or interpretation.

**Fourfold Hermeneutic**

Medieval thinkers – such as St. Augustine and Thomas Aquinas – held that there are four levels of interpretation with four distinct hierarchies. These levels conflate into one symbol, which can be read at any level, but ideally it should be read at all levels.

The first level is most commonly called 'the literal' and is exactly that – the literal interpretation of the symbol. So continuing our Saturn/Ascendant image above, Saturn rules the teeth (and skin and hair and skeleton, etc.), and the Ascendant rules the body; so when a transit of Saturn happens on our client's Ascendant, we might expect there to be some damage or negative impact from the malefic nature of Saturn to those areas.

The next level of interpretation is called 'the allegorical'. This is the use of metaphor, when we say one thing to mean another but we add something more to the subject by using the comparison. For example: 'I have bitten off more than I can chew'. The additional meaning attributed to the symbolic reading is that I might have allowed this to happen, and choices turned into consequences.

The following level of meaning is referred to as 'the tropological level', which means the point at which the symbol 'turns' into meaning something completely different from what was thought before. The word tropological derives from 'tropos' which means to turn. This turn is the colliding of the inner and outer worlds of human experience, when synchronicity happens, when we attribute a coincidence to have greater and more personal meaning than would otherwise normally be the case. For example, on the way to the dentist to fix the tooth, the client opened her purse to show the dentist the piece of tooth, and out popped her tax consultant's card. In that moment, a connection is made between the tooth and the tax consultant. Coincidentally, Saturn also rules tax consultants.

The final and most important move through the interpretation of this symbolism is the attainment of the next level which is 'the anagogical level', which implies a deeper understanding of the turn of the events that allows for a spiritual awakening or an adjustment of behaviour that is both morally correct, and appropriate to the situation as a whole. This is the point at which the client asks herself if her tax affairs are in order, if they truly and morally reflect her lifestyle and integrity, and if there is any financial imbalance in her life, which could be causing her to feel that she is overwhelmed or overly burdened. She then considers what she might be able to do to remedy that without impacting negatively on others and with an appreciation of karma in the widest sense of the word.

Here we can see how the symbol – the astrological signature of Saturn/Ascendant – has moved through all levels. The fourfold hermeneutic is a useful way to consider our signatures then. We trace the movement of the interpretation of the signature from the literal to the allegorical, from allegorical to tropological, tropological to anagogical.

In his book *The Moment of Astrology*, Geoffrey Cornelius introduces the 'The Fourfold Hermeneutic of Medieval Christianity' as a model for astrologers to understand the various levels on which symbolism can be interpreted in the natal chart. He suggests that this model, which is based on Origen's accounts of the miracles in biblical texts, is coded both into astrology and our DNA as humans: we seek to transcend the physical, literal, and corporeal world and to transform through revelation into a more collective, meaningful union with the divine. By linking the fourfold hermeneutic with the astrological chart, Cornelius puts the human being in the natal chart back into the whole world, not just the physical world, but back into the world of soul – back into cosmos. The fourfold hermeneutic thus becomes a story for everyone to live and participate in.

We locate ourselves in it, and we live it through all the axes of the cross in the natal chart.

This hermeneutic move is not exclusive to astrology nor to orthodox religions per se, but is available to the whole host of psychodynamic therapists who treat people in pain. The central question in this hermeneutic is: 'What does this mean to (or for) myself and my soul's path?' Using the literal events in the life of the patient as being symbolic of something else – so that these events become an allegory or metaphor, and unfolding the metaphor in such a way as to present alternate options to the default actions or behaviour of the patient going forward – can be considered a fourfold hermeneutic move of a Christian or divinatory order.

This is where I, personally, consider astrology to be divinatory: symbolic interpretation of signatures in a chart lead to the soulful, healing transformation of a patient. Astrology can be seen as a symbolic language, but without the participation of the client, and more importantly, *without the co-creating of narrative*, it is a semantic exercise, not divination. Barbara Tedlock asserts that the definition of 'divination' incorporates or implies the participation of an interpreter, a voice that allows the symbolic to speak.[96] That role is ours. So, while we work through the signatures or asterisms in this chapter, I ask that we hold that thought of the fourfold hermeneutic, that signatures are both literal and figurative (sometimes simultaneously) and contradictory to be sure, but with careful interpretation, with one eye on the physical plane and the other on the cosmos, the astrologer can help find meaning for the client's experience of their personal narrative.

**Prominent Signatures**

One of the issues that continues to raise its ugly head is that of empowerment within the relationship. Financial inequality nearly always has a direct bearing if the woman in question is vulnerable. It seems conception is always more likely if the 'nest is secure'. One of the reasons why a woman might find herself in a financially unequal situation is that she might have been trying seek financial independence in the first place, and finds herself in a double bind when trying to conceive.

So the first signature is that of a 10th house luminary. Either the Sun or the Moon in the 10th house is likely to suggest someone whose core identity or desire is to be in the public sphere, or to express their solar energy in a public role or leadership position. Such a woman will usually leave it to the last minute to have a family, as she is aware somehow that she cannot have both at the same time. Someone with a strong desire to be an important cog in the wheel of society will not easily be able to give up that avenue of self-expression in the course of having a family, whose demands are direct competition to her core essence and personal sense of fulfilment. A frank discussion about childcare and acknowledging the importance of a career to this woman can help prepare her for parenthood. Expectations about this process are best laid out fairly early on, so that the fear of losing independence does not psychologically inhibit conception.

The next broad signature in both male and female charts is a truly damaged Saturn – cadent, retrograde, besieged, no essential dignity. This spells more trouble if aspecting the Moon. Moon/Saturn contacts in medieval works are nearly always interpreted as being negative, and curiously, there is little actually said about it relating to fertility per se, but there are references to the condition of the mother in these charts as being compromised either in health or in social standing – either sick or a slave.[97] This point is valid when assessing modern charts – if one's mother's path to parenthood was not an easy transition, how would it affect your own? Memories from childhood richly inform us on deep levels of the difficulties of nurturing children at the expense of personal development. Such mothers might be deeply resentful of the sacrifices that had to be made, some might bear physical scars, some might just be negligent, unable to be emotionally intimate, some might just be overly strict. Whatever the manifestation, there will be some overtone as to how your client experienced nurturing and if they have confidence in being able to nurture in return. Feelings of self-worth are brought into focus, and there might be guilt associated with failure to conceive, with a popular narrative being 'I am struggling to conceive, perhaps I don't deserve a child' or worse, 'I had a termination once, now I am being punished'.

There might be a fear with Moon/Saturn hard aspects that they will repeat negative parenting patterns. Using astrology you might be able to overcome this thinking by demonstrating that in a family of multiple children, each child might be born with a different 4th/10th house axis, and therefore they will each experience their parents differently. This helps your client appreciate that whatever their own parents did is always seen through a certain lens of this axis, and so reality has little to do with how one feels about mother/father. This model not only provides an opportunity for healing old hurts, it also instantly gets the hopeful mum off the hook somewhat, allowing her to see her relationships with her future children in healthy new ways. This is a powerful tool in fertility astrology – giving women (and men) permission to be less than perfect parents.

On a physical level (in women in particular) the Moon/Saturn hard aspect brings its own problems. Ridder-Patrick states:

> Like Sun-Saturn, Moon-Saturn afflictions can show up as hereditary diseases, but the most common pathology is neurosis and depression owing to the fear and abnormal sensitivity that Saturn produces when aspecting the Moon. It gives a slowed and inhibited emotional response as well as restrictive and controlling eating behaviours, which provide fertile ground for illness of all kinds.[98]

This bears out what I have noticed in my practice about this signature being an indicator of the narrative of 'not enough' in my client's experience of life – as in, not enough blood supply in the uterus to support a conception, not enough hormone to sustain pregnancy after implantation, not enough eggs, not enough money or resources, not enough time (age-related) and, finally, not enough space – literally in the uterus (bicornate uterus, for example).

When Ridder-Patrick states that Moon/Saturn 'is associated with chronic disturbances in the water balance, defects of mucus membranes and bladder diseases', I think of the role of cervical mucus – too little mucus at ovulation means that fertilisation is more difficult, as the sperm need to swim up through the mucus into the uterine cavity, and the mucus should not be too acidic, otherwise it will kill the very sperm it is trying to bring into the uterus. Saturn is often associated with fungal infections such as Candida, which also inhibit fertilisation and are common in women with this signature.

In addition, Moon/Saturn in women 'can be linked with late onset of puberty, and with late, painful or scant menstruation.'[99] Thus, low ovarian reserve and problems with thickening of the lining of the uterus are both echoed here. There is also a condition known as PCOS, which is polycystic ovarian syndrome. Women with this syndrome often present with ovarian cysts (which occur when the outer lining of the egg is too hard to burst on ovulation; this prevents the release of the hormones necessary to stimulate the next stage of fertilisation or menstruation), acne and other skin complaints such as skin tags on the underarm and breast area, facial hair, thinning of hair or baldness on head, heavy bleeding with menstruation, and more.

On an emotional level of interpretation, these women can be described as 'defensive' and they have 'defensive eggs' which need assisted fertilisation as the hard outer lining makes it difficult for the sperm to penetrate naturally. A process called ICSI is often employed to force a fertilisation in these cases. To most astrologers reading these lists of symptoms the connection with Saturn is quite obvious – skin, hair, and boundaries of eggs being the common theme. So a women whose complexion is dark (Moon = complexion) or whose Ascendant is Saturn (either rising or actually in the 1st house) might just present with this problem, which can be addressed on an emotional level in an inquiry about why her eggs are so defensive.

I am not suggesting for a minute that these physical symptoms and others are magically and easily overcome by a little light therapy. On the contrary. But it is possible to change patterning in younger women if they are caught in their twenties and not in their forties. Too few eggs is common enough in women trying to conceive after thirty-five, and this can be overcome with drug therapies or donor egg programs if necessary. A woman born with a bi-cornate uterus or septum can have this repaired with a relatively small procedure and with good result. Hormone therapy can assist with maintaining pregnancy once implantation has occurred, but blood supply can be tricky and new techniques involving Viagra are proving to be helpful in thickening the lining of the uterus.[100] Personally, I find this latest treatment most interesting since a lot of my charts with this affliction frequently present a Moon/Saturn/Uranus aspect pattern (in the past seven years, the age of my client base has been mostly those born in the mid 1960s with the Saturn/Uranus opposition in their natal charts), and this signature could be astrologically defined as an emasculating personality type, whose functioning can result in denial of their own femininity and consequently their uteri reject embryos due to a lack of receptive conditions. The treatment of Viagra in males is to restore a man's physical masculinity, and the same would seem to be true for women – increasing the blood flow to the uterus makes the uterus more receptive to conception. Perhaps the signature for Saturn/Uranus/Moon or Sun should read: truncation of, disassociation of, denial of the reproductive principle in both males and females. This is very reminiscent of the Uranus myth.

In my practice, a lot of older women (over forty) have eventually resorted to having hysterectomies (the removal of the uterus entirely) usually leaving the ovaries intact to continue endocrine function, for a number of different reasons, ranging from physical (heavy bleeding with menstruation, fibroids, or endometriosis) to psychosomatic (irritation with the inconvenience of a menstrual cycle after childbearing years, resistance to aging, extending a healthy sexual life and to eliminate the risk of cervical or uterine cancers). This fear of aging or fear of cancers associated with reproductive organs is a perfectly sound signature for Saturn/Moon on its own, and a potential risk for those with charts with this signature.

In a male chart, Moon/Saturn contacts might be descriptive of the relationship he has with his own wife/mother and other females in his family, the message being, 'fear the feminine, it does not nourish, it devours', or that emotional realms are hard to access, and belong to the wife and not to him personally. I have often seen men with this signature and infertility issues choose women who seem to be predisposed to being depressive or postnatally depressive types, who have emotional difficulties quite separate from the male chart altogether. It would seem as though these men have so thoroughly and effectively projected their Moons onto the nearest female that any attempt to get them to own it might seem futile in the quest for fertility, but it is well worth the investigation in regular therapy. Sometimes this signature in men produces (literal) fear around financial security, which is at the heart of the matter, and they might even withhold financial support for IVF, which is Saturn personified at his most self-destructive and self-limiting best.

Of course, hormone function is one of the most important functions for fertility for both males and females. In females the hormones FSH and LSH are regulated by the hypothalamus and the endocrine system to thicken the lining of the endometrium and to ovulate and release eggs ready for fertilisation each month. Without a functioning hormone system fertilisation will not happen, and women who suffer from deficiencies can be treated with chemical hormones most successfully. In males, the same hormones FSH and LSH function in a similar fashion to produce spermatozoa in the testicles. Testosterone is manufactured and regulated by the hypothalamus in order to both produce sperm and to maintain sexual characteristics (facial hair, pubic hair and deepening of voice, etc.) during puberty.

Aristotle showed the most profound understanding of the role of hormones in fertility when he declared that children are born from the head of man.[101] He meant literally that desire – sexual desire in particular – is the prime motivator of fertility because of the active role that men play in the sexual act, and because desire arrives (albeit a split second) before an erection. It therefore seemed reasonable to Aristotle that desire originated in the brain of men. In this statement, he also reveals his understanding of hormone function; even though he could not 'see' or observe hormones in the blood, he still had an idea that this 'pnuema', or hormone/pheromone, animated the soul to procreate, and because of the location of the organ – the hypothalamus – at the base of the skull, he asserted that this was the origin of sperm. And Aristotle has been proved correct insomuch as the hormones released by this gland at the base of the head of both females and males, plays a pivotal (one could say primal) role in the production of both sperm and the hormones required to regulate the menstrual cycle and the release of eggs in females.

Aristotle's concept of pneuma is extended here, inasmuch as the hormone is undetectable, and the yearning or desire for children is formed in the brain and not the sexual organ itself. Yet the hormone animates the cellular process of reproduction from this place of yearning, or desire. It is precisely this yearning that gives life, that animates the physical to achieve the elusive successful conception. It could be interpreted astrologically as a Neptune function – which is entirely congruent with what astrologers currently believe – that Neptune co-rules the endocrine system and the liver function along with Jupiter.

Neptune is also the planet associated with depression and addictions and with the process of falling in love – animating the soul in a way to ensure procreation. Ridder-Patrick cites Mars/Neptune as a marker for autoimmune disorders, loss of the ability to fight off infection, or to discharge pus. I would extend this interpretation to include toxic blood disorders such as HIV, as well as sexually addictive behaviours and STIs.

This has been called the pathological aspect because Mars, the warrior of the body's defences, is confused and undermined by Neptune's diffuseness and lack of boundaries. The body does not know whether to attack or to surrender and while it is paralysed, trying to make up its mind, infection sets up home at whichever site provides the best breeding ground. The result can be chronic, hard to diagnose, low-grade infections. There can be paralysis, weakness or wasting of the muscles, and a great susceptibility to autoimmune disorders, where the body is attacked by its own defence system.[102]

One autoimmune condition that presents is called 'killer cell' syndrome, which is when the female uterus rejects or fails to let the embryo implant as it senses that the embryo is foreign. The immune system responds in an overly dramatic fashion to this intrusion and literally kills the embryo. This can be difficult to get a handle on, as the only indicator could be frequent failed IVF cycles in spite of the embryo being in good condition, and the hormone blood readings perfect, and all other indicators fine. Clients with this signature report other general symptoms such as allergies to various foods, alcohol and/or medications, sensitivities to textiles (itchy label syndrome), or huge addictions to drugs or alcohol or smoking. The over-riding factor seems to best described as an increased sensitivity to the environment coupled with poor boundaries and the tendency to give in, or give up, when resistance is met (by the physical body or on a more esoteric level). It is also common to find a diagnosis of anemia among my female clients with this signature.

In male infertility charts, Neptune with Mars in hard aspect can present with problems of impotency, sometimes only temporarily during the time of trying to conceive, which possibly indicates a deeper desire to renounce the path of parenting, or a possible addiction to the sexual act itself, in which case the sperm material could be infected from contact with STIs. Then there is the issue of impotency, where the hormone responsible for shutting off the valve at the base of the penis to sustain an erection malfunctions and, as a result, the blood flows into the penis and flows out again. Other manifestations in male charts of this signature include what I call the 'monk's signature' – that is the sublimation of the sexual in favour of the spiritual and the renunciation of the result of the sexual, i.e. children. This is especially true when the opposition or conjunction happens in the 5th or 11th house. If these men do have a change of heart and decide to marry, and try for a family, this signature will often manifest as a poor libido; there could be long periods of abstinence, and a high level of stress caused by their desire to conceive naturally rather than through assisted treatments. This could be an unbearable pressure and result in couples (or men) simply giving up, throwing in the towel all too soon. These are men whose philosophy regarding pregnancy and conception is: what will be, will be, God decides, I will not interfere with the process. It is a very passive position, a defensive one, and entirely understandable in the context of the perspective of their chart.

The Stoics took this concept a step further and suggested that different types of pneuma are responsible for keeping things hanging together coherently, so that the physical body is held in a tension between the outer and the inner world; and that this boundary is constantly re-adjusting itself to maintain a balance in order to differentiate between those worlds. This concept of boundary issues is also extremely representative of Neptune. We are all too familiar with the concept of escapism, and the desire to return to the Matrix of all there is and the yearning of some heavily Piscean charts to merge with the entire collective. And astrologers are equally aware of the toxic result that follows weakened boundaries, softened defence systems, immune disorders, etc. So it follows then that charts with heavy Neptune contacts to the Ascendant, Moon, Sun, or Almuten of Pregnancy are also tinged with this contradiction – the yearning for, but also the renunciation of children. These charts seem to represent a life spent in the emotional space of earning/addiction/desire, so that successful conception in the case of fertility astrology, may seem unlikely in the context of a chart whose narrative is that of yearning and not used to getting desires met, but living constantly in that desire of and experiencing the lack of success as renunciation (or victimhood). A lot of my female clients with an angular Neptune suffer from some fantasy element in their narratives, and this fantasy can be played out in their refusal (in some cases) to seek proper or appropriate treatment, all the while hoping against the odds that they will fall pregnant naturally, and the usual excuses are: not wanting to take the drugs required for treatment as they are 'toxic' and 'unnatural', or having a religious or spiritual attitude that is incongruent with IVF, or having a general distrust of western modern medicine and hospitals. Superstitions are rife in this field. By not seeking out the treatments appropriate for their personal situations, they will not fall pregnant, thereby allowing them to live out and manifest the 'martyr' or 'victim' aspect of Neptune.

Charts with Neptune to Saturn – this is generational, so only planets in tight orb to angles and luminaries really count – seem to present with the issue of not getting the thing that is desired, and the experience of loss or the renunciation of something that was once so treasured. The physical experience seems to be that the endocrine system is under stress or limitation, so that there is not enough hormone to sustain the desire for the precious baby or pregnancy. Saturn/Neptune by transit or solar arc is thus also a strong signifier of miscarriage due to a lack of hormones to sustain the pregnancy.

Another hormone common to both sexes – prolactin – plays an important role in males. In females, prolactin is responsible for the production of breast milk. In males, prolactin is released after ejaculation. It represses the effect of dopamine, which is partly responsible for sexual arousal, thus causing the male's refractory period. Researchers at the University of Paisley and the Technische Hochschule Zürich have recently discovered that prolactin provides the body with sexual gratification after sexual acts.[103] High levels of prolactin are found in males who suffer from infertility related to sperm count and morphology. These men are also prone to present with feminine body shape and texture – rounded, fleshy and bald. Unusually high amounts are suspected to be responsible for impotence and loss of libido. Robert Winston is not, however, entirely convinced by the medical or biologically scientific explanation, even though he acknowledges the correlation between the high levels found in men with fertility issues. He suggests that:

> High levels may occasionally be caused by a benign tumour of the pituitary which is easily treatable by minor surgery. The evidence that prolactin really affects sperm production is extremely poor.[104]

I find it difficult to believe that the correlation between high levels of prolactin in men with fertility issues is merely arbitrary. I would suggest that this condition is a really good indicator for an astrological signature of Moon/Mars in male charts, further suggesting a psychosocial dynamic responsible for infertility as opposed to a biological and medically treatable condition.

In male charts the Moon/Mars signature seems to appear with the most regularity in men whose sperm is tested for poor morphology. There are three conditions that apply to sperm for the effectiveness of fertilisation :

Morphology – the shape of the sperm
Motility – the movement of the sperm
Count – the number of sperm per cc of fluid

There can be few sperm, or low motility, but the morphology is the one thing that has to be right for natural fertilisation to occur.

The main function of morphology appears to be that the head of the spermatozoa has a cap on it, which on meeting the egg, sloughs off and releases an enzyme that softens the lining of the egg in order to facilitate penetration of the sperm into the egg. Once a single sperm has approached an egg in this way, no other sperm is able to penetrate. Twin births are mostly a result of two different eggs being fertilised and confined at the same time, or a single-cell zygote that splits into two separate embryos.

Sperm is replenished every seventy-two days or so, which means that every three months the quality of the sperm could be different due to a variety of factors which are not entirely understood by science. Several theories suggest that alcohol abuse, drug abuse, stress, and smoking all take their toll on the quality of sperm. Until fairly recently it was thought that it was only eggs that aged, but new studies show that sperm quality does decline with age and that older sperm has the same tendency to produce chromosomal disorders as older eggs.

In male charts, Moon/Mars aspects highlight potentially emasculating relationships with women, anger directed at mother figures or inwardly shameful feelings regarding sexuality, unresolved issues of substituting sex (or habitual masturbation) for real emotional intimacy. On the physical it manifests as the inability of the sperm to penetrate the egg, and consequently fertilisation does not occur. Unless sperm is tested at a reliable laboratory, this will not be obvious; no indication in colour, viscosity or volume of seminal fluid is of relevance. Hard aspects of Mars to Moon therefore can be interpreted as a physical challenge in the form of too many female hormones, or an emotional challenge of intense relationships with women that result in feelings of anger, emasculation, or humiliation.

Interestingly the absence of Sirius from the night sky, which in

Egyptian calendars marks the beginning of the period of mourning of Isis, is the same length of time as it takes for a man to replenish his stock of sperm, give or take a few hours, which further entrenches this star and this constellation as a fertile narrative. What makes this useful to astrologers and therapists is that if a man with such a signature can come to a therapy to concentrate solely on this aspect of his relationship with his mother and women – i.e. the potential for emasculation in his chart and the effect on his developing sexuality as a young teenager – then he has a really good chance of changing the nature and quality of his sperm. In this day and age we are familiar with the concept of mind over matter and the ability of therapy to shift paradigms and grow souls, so it is not an entirely foreign concept to expect that the quality of sperm can change within a three-month period of intense therapy.[105] In female charts Moon/Mars often presents as surgery to reproductive organs or breasts at some stage, surgery to pierce ovarian cysts and appendectomies, or through invasive fertility treatments such as ICSI, where the egg gets forcibly fertilised. Ridder-Patrick notes that 'Moon-Mars represents the mobilisation of emotions. An everyday example of this is blushing.'[106] In my practice, the phrase 'mobilisation of emotions' is sometimes at the root of the problem; feelings of inadequacy fuelled by competiveness can make women struggling to conceive even angrier (usually directed at other women), leading to terminal resentment. This signature can be 'associated with copious menstruation, bilious and nausea, and fevers that produce reddish skin eruptions'.[107] Further, Ridder-Patrick states, 'Reinhold Ebertin links the combination with involuntary muscle movement, thyroid gland function, and Grave's disease'.[108] In my experience, termination of pregnancy, either voluntary or by miscarriage, or the disinclination to have children, may also be found with this aspect.

**Moon through the Signs with the Moon as a Signifier for the Eggs, Ovaries and Uterus**

**ARIES:** Ovulation tends to be earlier in the cycle than in other signs, so natural conception might be difficult if one is waiting for day fourteen before sexual activity. Ovulation can happen as early as day eight or nine, and ultrasound scans and blood tests can verify this. A more accurate assessment of when ovulation is likely to happen can assist in natural conceptions. Women with an Aries Moon are often impatient and this needs to be taken into consideration when advising them on timing. They will not be able to wait six months to try, so you may have to 'dig deep' and find them a potentially lucky time sooner rather than later, and you will have to alert them to the fact that although this is not the best or optimum time, it is better to try with a small lucky transit rather than leaving them to try on their own at an unlucky time. Because of the early ovulation, follicles can be undeveloped, and as a consequence no fertilisation happens.

**TAURUS**: The Moon is in exaltation in Taurus, which can be interpreted as 'promises but does not deliver'.[109] Taurus is a fixed sign, so the egg might have a hard outer lining, preventing natural fertilisation of the egg to form an embryo. Larger doses of pharmaceuticals are needed to stimulate ovulation as Taurus is a stubborn sign and subtle treatment is sometimes not effective. Unexplained infertility is often linked to the Moon in Taurus as the eggs look good on examination and at fertilisation, the embryos can be A grade, but still not implant, so careful examination of all endocrine function including that of progesterone after implantation needs to be managed. Women with Moon in Taurus also show a predisposition to PCOS – a condition that means that ovarian cysts and issues to do with the release of the egg at ovulation make conception difficult. One popular manifestation of the Moon in Taurus is that the cycle is sometimes longer than average, and in some cases up to ninety days.

**GEMINI**: Gemini is traditionally a barren sign, being an air sign. It is also a young, androgynous sign ruled by Mercury, so issues to do with egg maturation and follicle forming are obstacles for those with the Moon in Gemini. These women produce eggs, but sometimes without a follicle, and if they do fertilise with IVF, the cell multiplication is slower than usual or the embryo forms at a rate that is not normal and with the possible consequence of not making it to transfer stage. These women also sometimes present with scanty, light periods and therefore the lining of the uterus is too thin, making implantation difficult to achieve. Both Gemini rising and Gemini Moon has the added problem of being either so stressed or so scattered that the lining of the uterus does not thicken adequately. Telling a Gemini to relax, or take time off work, is not typically effective; they will simply fill the vacuum with another stressful activity.

Rather encourage them to have acupuncture, or to remain at work but meditate briefly in between appointments, focusing on visualisations (which engage the mind in a different way).

**CANCER**: The Moon rules Cancer, a water sign, so all looks really good for egg production and the uterus. The only downside with this signature is the emotional investment is sometimes really difficult for these women. They frequently voice their fear of not getting pregnant, or they find the process of fertility treatment emotionally draining. The astrologer simply needs to reassure them that this is normal and to support them emotionally, so that they don't give up too soon. Ovulation is good, sometimes more than one egg at a time, so if they are going for IVF they will produce many eggs for retrieval and are often able to freeze embryos or participate in egg share schemes, which satisfies them on a different and completely unexpected level.

**LEO**: Leo is also a traditionally barren sign, but, considering the technology at our disposal, it would be crass to write off whole signs as infertile. Yet the traditional observation is still valid in light of Leo being a fixed, fire sign. PCOS is common in women with the Moon in Leo, as inflammation at ovulation is often a condition linked to fire signs. Endocrine function needs to be observed for any variation from the norm, and if the Moon is in any way linked to Mars or Saturn, or Pluto, the occurrence of possible ectopic pregnancies is indicated.

**VIRGO**: The Moon in Virgo has issues with procrastination, so these women will delay pregnancy until 'all the boxes are ticked'. Their fussiness regarding diet, allergies and such, may mean that they are not getting the nutrients they actually need, or that they are genuinely allergic to their husband's sperm, quite literally. Women with a Virgo Moon might have issues to do with maturation of follicles in the eggs as the ruler of the Moon is Mercury, which has an androgynous quality to it. Virgo Moon and Virgo rising people can be highly strung and exhibit OCD behaviours, which might mean that the lining of the uterus is not thick enough at implantation. Hyperstimulation is not indicated unless there is a hard aspect from Jupiter, and ovulation will be within the normal standard range in terms of regularity and reliability.

**LIBRA**: The Moon in Libra manifests in fertility charts as eggs or embryos that look great, but do not implant or result in conception. The rulership of Venus is tricky as it leads one to assume that this signature is fertile and benefic, but the air element seems to keep this quality in the realm of concept and not in physical form. Moon in Libra presents with vagueness; the growth of the follicle may be immature, and sometimes ovulation might not happen at all during the cycle. The lining of the uterus can be on the thin side, and not 'moist' enough in the astrological sense. Psychologically, Moon in Libra often views nurturing as a concept. Unnecessary levels of perfection are projected onto the idea of motherhood, leaving the woman permanently doubting whether she is 'worthy' enough to be a mother, or if she can satisfy unrealistic goals of becoming the perfect mother. She might even have idealised her own nurturing experience, and this could also feed this unhelpful narrative. Also, the common indecisiveness associated with the Sun in Libra applies to the Moon in this sign. All individuals with this signature could delay child-rearing until too late, or abandon it altogether, in their quest for the perfect mate, the perfect time, and the perfect circumstances.

**SCORPIO**: The Moon is in detriment in Scorpio, so the quality of the eggs are in question with this signature. Alleviating aspects from Jupiter may help, but if your client is nearing forty years of age, a conversation about 'donor egg' might need to happen sooner rather than later. This signature also presents with heavy bleeding with menstruation, PCOS (especially if Scorpio rising) and the eggs might need ICSI due to the 'fixed' nature of Scorpio. Detriment might also refer to fertilisation happening out of the mainstream, possibly reflecting the need for aggressive medical treatment, such as IVF. Ovarian cysts are common with this sign, and excess mucus at ovulation might swamp the fallopian tubes, rather than assist the flow of the embryo gently into the uterus. Infections (due to inflammation) of the fallopian tubes are indicated if Mercury is involved by aspect. On a psychological note, the deep-seated resentment that the Moon in Scorpio can hold might be preventing a conception. Gentle reminders about letting go of the past (which may or may not include a termination due to an early surprise pregnancy) can help ease the situation and make for a more positive, optimistic approach. Scorpio Moons have a tendency (in my practice at least) to be the most negative, and fall into the trap of reading too many internet articles that are doom and gloom, and identify only with the harshest of outcomes. Feelings of guilt and of being undeserving are especially highlighted for women with Moon in Scorpio.

**SAGITTARIUS**: Happy-go-lucky Moon in Sagittarius needs very little encouragement to produce large quantities of eggs. Ruled by Jupiter, this is the signature that most suffers from hyperstimulation – a painful and dangerous event if not managed properly. Egg quantity is not a problem for this signature, and neither is quality. Ovulation is normal, menstruation can be heavy, but not painful, and the lining of the uterus is thick and healthy unless other aspects mitigate and threaten this fortunate Moon. A further complication of this Moon is that the lining of the uterus might 'wander', and endometriosis can occur. This Moon sign is also the 'eternal optimist', and some might delay child-bearing thinking they have all the time in the world, and their appetite for experience might lead them to procrastinate.

**CAPRICORN**: Moon in Capricorn is typically 'stingy' and produces just enough eggs, but no abundance. Sometimes the eggs need ICSI to facilitate fertilisation, as Capricorn is a sign most often associated with excellent boundaries, so the eggs have a defensive layer of enzyme that the sperm finds difficult to penetrate. The lining of the uterus tends to be too thin – again a function of the stinginess of Capricorn. Treatments such as acupuncture have shown to help in these cases. The Moon is also psychologically compromised in this sign. Issues to do with nurturing and love received and given might cause the woman to delay, or even avoid intimacy and ultimately pregnancy. Submitting to pregnancy – and all the vulnerabilities that go hand in hand with the process of becoming a mother – overwhelm the Moon in Capricorn and this might be a further stumbling block. Fear of loss of financial support, fear of not having enough 'resources' might also contribute to the inability to yield to the process.

**AQUARIUS**: Aquarius Moons are the most difficult to interpret, as there is so much that is unpredictable about them. Surprise pregnancies in spite of using contraception are common, as well as irregular ovulation cycles – either scanty or irregular menstruation, but also the capacity to ovulate at different times each month. Sometimes ovulation happens on day nine, sometimes on day sixteen, sometimes not at all. That is why the pregnancies are sometimes a surprise if one is using natural contraception, such as the rhythm method. Careful charting is necessary if your client is trying to conceive naturally, as you don't want to exhaust the couple by making them have sex every other day. They need to understand how to anticipate ovulation so that they can minimise the damage they do to their sexual relationship in the long run. This signature also indicates that there might be a septum in the uterus, or a 'bi-cornate' uterus, which is divided into two chambers. This condition can cause issues with implantation and premature births, but there are surgical solutions that are relatively minor and successful in repairing the uterus.

**PISCES**: As Jupiter rules the Moon in Pisces, one can expect a higher quantity of eggs at ovulation than average. However, the nature of Pisces is not so transparent, things are not always what they seem, so care needs to be taken when making the judgement that the eggs are going to be perfect just because the Moon is ruled by Jupiter.

### The Moon and the Outer Planets

It is useful to have a sense of the Moon's relationship to Uranus, Neptune, and Pluto. The following paragraphs rely on Ridder-Patrick's research on how these outer planets affect the Moon.

**Moon/Uranus**: Ridder-Patrick makes the case for irregular ovulation in her interpretation of Moon/Uranus:

> There can be menstrual irregularities, pain at ovulation and dysmenorrhea. It can lead to colic in any fluid-excreting or fluid containing organ… Wherever Uranus is involved it is common to want to over-ride the restrictions of the natural cycles of the body. I have known women with these aspects who can, at will, put back the arrival of a period.[110]

In my practice women with this signature often ovulate on different days each month, making it difficult to track when trying to conceive naturally. These same women might also experience surprise pregnancies, or very erratic IVF cycles, where sometimes things go very wrong or very right, but with no reliability.

**Moon/Neptune:** Charts with Moon/Neptune contacts are especially tricky since the role of the mother is under the spotlight once more, but this time her role is not so easily defined as it was with Moon/Saturn and the concept of 'not having enough'. This time she could be an alcoholic, she could be an absent yoga teacher, she could be on anti-depressants, or she could be a really talented painter/musician or muse. Or she could seem so perfect, that any attempt to be a mother herself could be too overwhelming, or the concept of mothering could be the holy grail itself – all too intangible, all too seemingly impossible to achieve – in which case the only outcome is denial of the experience of mothering altogether in the face of certain failure.

I have seen male charts with Moon/Neptune presenting with toxicity of the genetic material itself – namely the sperm. This signature has presented before in charts where both males or females have had chemotherapy as a result of cancer or childhood leukaemia. These charts are seriously challenged and success depends on whether or not sperm was frozen before treatment commenced – whether the male was old enough to be producing sperm at all, or whether or not the female is willing to try using donor eggs. Freezing eggs to be used later in life is a relatively new innovation; many of my clients have not had the benefit of this technology. Where any cryotherapy (freezing of eggs or sperm) is involved, Neptune usually is too. Indeed, even Dr. Silberman, the man who developed this technique, has a Moon/Neptune signature in his natal chart.

The overall interpretation of this aspect is that there are complications with diagnosis as the patient is confused with boundary issues, has psychosomatic problems and/or conflicting medical results of tests leading to doctors being unable to treat for any particular affliction, in the light of no symptoms. In my experience, this aspect signifies that there is some unknown quantity in the egg production, and ovulation. Neptune hints at substance abuse or recreational drug use, or even environmental pollution issues that may or may not have an impact on the quality of the eggs, or it may just be that there is a chromosomal irregularity where missing DNA might mean that the egg is of poor quality and will not produce viable embryos after fertilisation. Egg donor recipients in my database mostly have hard Moon/Neptune aspects. The client will not know for sure if this is the case until they have tried repeated IVF and had many transfers not resulting in a viable pregnancy. This means that while they might have a positive pregnancy test, the embryo may not develop, and no heartbeat is detected at six weeks.

In the context of IVF and other innovative technologies, the only factor that remains 'unknown' or nearly impossible to diagnose from screening or blood tests ahead of time, is the quality of the egg. Only after ruling out all other factors will the medical specialist recommend PGN testing (a test geneticists do on the embryo), but this means sacrificing a few embryos and one round of IVF, which is costly both financially and emotionally. Where there is a strong hard Moon/Neptune aspect this potential needs to be mentioned and explored, as a donor egg might be the only route to motherhood for your client.

Often clients with this aspect also have unrealistic expectations regarding motherhood and nurturing, and project fantasy elements onto their partners, their own mothers, and the process of how they are going to achieve pregnancy in the first place. These clients are often deeply distressed that they are in the position of having to have treatment at all. They far prefer the 'magical' romantic version, where they conceive spontaneously on their wedding anniversary after a candle-lit dinner. They are so fanatical about this, they can even 'imagine' a few pregnancies along the way, so careful monitoring of the actual medical landscape is required to get a clearer picture of what is really happening and what the client thinks is happening. There is no judgement here. These clients are just expressing themselves in the only way they know how, and gentle handling of them is required so that they don't lose hope entirely.

Neptune (in modern rulerships) and Jupiter rule the liver/metabolic processes and the endocrine system, and as such, disorders like diabetes can contribute to infertility inasmuch as they interfere with the hormone regulation of the menstrual cycle and the maturation of sperm in males. Neptune with Venus indicates a 'sweet tooth' and if diabetes has not been diagnosed yet, your client should at least be aware of the potential in the future. As Neptune is associated with pharmaceuticals and other recreational drugs, it should be noted that sometimes the presence of Neptune configured with the Moon and Venus just might indicate that the client, at some point in their lives, might embark on a phase of pharmaceutical treatment.

**Moon/Pluto**: Pluto nearly always brings trauma, upheavals, and a good dose of destruction. My clients have reported a recent death in the family, loss of money or the physical home, renovations to home, loss of friends or partners, or ill health. The 'bad' things do not have to happen to the client directly, so it is useful to ask questions to understand if other people in their charts are at the receiving end of her Pluto transit, before leaping in and making dire predictions that will further devastate a woman who is struggling to conceive. In terms of physical manifestation, Ridder-Patrick states:

> The most common problems that I have found in women are fibroids, endometriosis and excessive menstrual bleeding. Many of these patients, whatever the aspect, have either had or been threatened with a hysterectomy or have intense and sometimes difficult experiences around childbirth where the survival of the mother or child or both was at risk. There is also a link with disturbances of bowel function and surgical removal of parts of the colon, which in some cases ends with a colostomy. Eating disorders like anorexia are another possibility, often in an attempt to control the body's demands to mature, ripen and become sexual. Moon-Pluto contacts are also associated with life-threatening conditions like cancer, especially of the bowel and reproductive organs.
>
> During treatment some patients start to acknowledge an uncanny degree of intuitive insight and power that they had been afraid to look at before because they felt overwhelmed by it. Once the psychological element was recognised, with astrological counselling, and the realisation that they were not mad or bad, the physical problems lessened and became more manageable.[111]

Pluto will also tax the adrenal glands, which will in turn affect the endocrine system, as the 'fight or flight' mechanism is activated with this signature. The process of fertilisation is a Moon activity, so the presence of Pluto in hard aspect indicates that there might be overtones of trauma or fear in the fertilisation of the embryo; this could be a manifestation of the actual process of IVF which is very invasive, painful, and humiliating.

Or, there could be at the most negative end of the interpretation, a rape, an ectopic pregnancy, or life or death issues at births. *Do not alarm your client* by leaping in with these predictions as absolutes! Let them tell their stories, and take it from there.

**The Condition of Mercury**
With all fertility clients, and indeed with every young woman I see, I investigate the condition and dignity of Mercury carefully to establish the essential condition of her fallopian tubes. When I suggest that Mercury rules the fallopian tubes, it is not just because they are a 'way travelled' by the egg, or that the tubes 'connect' the ovaries with the uterus – this is an over-simplistic interpretation. On a deeper, alchemical level, the fallopian tube is the location of the sperm's fertilisation of the egg, the 'cosmic marriage' of the solar and lunar principle as sperm and egg. In this symbolism, Mercury facilitates the coming together of sperm and egg to form the embryo, which then travels to the uterus, which accepts or rejects the embryo. Thus if Mercury is in detriment, this location experiences some form of compromise.

There are two placements for Mercury to be in detriment (in Pisces and in Sagittarius), and consequently, approximately 16 percent of all charts have this placement. My practice informs me that this is reflected in the number of conceptions that occur outside of wedlock, age group, or ethnic group. This Mercury will also often be found in one or both charts of people in a LGBTQI+ relationship, where conception usually happens through medical intervention.

Mercury combust the Sun (and often in fire signs) is frequently present with ectopic pregnancies, where the embryo embeds itself in the fallopian tube and not in the uterus – a dangerous and life-threatening condition, which usually results in an emergency operation to remove the offending tube. A Mesopotamian interpretation of this combust placement could be that the conception takes place in 'the other place' – which is of course the only other place it could embed itself. Another more recent finding in my research is that this placement resulting in the conception happening in 'the other place' occurs with some regularity in the charts of those women who have opted to donate their own eggs, thereby fulfilling the criteria of 'the other place' being the uterus of another woman.

Mercury with Uranus most frequently indicates a laparoscopy (small incision to the abdomen to investigate or operate on the tube), and also suggests the potential for IVF treatment – fertilization through technology and surgery. It is important to remember that, as women, we are not finished with fertility once we have decided not to have children, or once we have finished having our children, or even once we have heading for menopause. Fertility is an ongoing relationship we have with our bodies, and issues that come later in life are still represented by signatures like Mercury/Uranus. Women with this signature might not have a laparoscopy to fall pregnant, but they might have one later in life, for treatment of other reproductive issues, such as endometriosis or a hysterectomy.

Mercury with Neptune has presented with damage to the fallopian tubes due to STIs picked up and not treated, for example Chlamydia, which is a silent disease and can appear after one episode of sexual activity. Another more literal interpretation is that the fallopian tubes are unable to facilitate the peristaltic movement in order to collect the egg from the ovary and to move the embryo down into the uterus. The fallopian tubes need to be agile and nimble, and any hard aspect from Neptune suggests a certain sluggishness or paralysis of the tube and an inability to function properly.

Mercury/Pluto hard aspects often indicate trauma to the fallopian tubes in the form of infection and inflammation from STIs and subsequent blockage or damage requiring treatment, or the employment of treatments such as GIFT or ZIFT which insert the sperm and egg directly into the tube without fertilising them first – like a forced introduction, so to speak. Ectopic pregnancies are also indicated and the possible removal of part of a tube or a whole tube. Women with this aspect also frequently have themselves sterilised through a process called tubal ligation where the tube is cut on both sides and tied off, preventing any egg and sperm from reaching the uterus. This is also found with women with Mercury/Uranus.

Mercury/Pluto also indicates obstruction to the functioning of the tube due to endometriosis, the growth of fibroids in and around the ovaries. There is a personal, and unique, interpretation for each and every placement of Mercury in a chart, and it would behove a fertility astrologer to carefully investigate this as a source of potentially helpful information that cannot be seen without medical intervention. Saving time in fertility treatment is part of the battle, when women are only starting to have families in their forties.

## Mercury through the Signs

**ARIES**: Fallopian tubes are robust, in full working order (not considering aspects), and the only danger lies in the impulsive nature of Aries – sexual activity without adequate protection can result in infections that scar the tissue, but this is not generally problematic unless indicated through combustion or poor condition.

**TAURUS**: Stubborn, lazy fallopian tubes which will not move around to pick up the egg, but delightfully moist and humid and hospitable for a travelling embryo.

**GEMINI**: Fallopian tubes that can adapt to current tides, turn inside out to accommodate a tricky travelling egg, and efficient in delivery of the newly fertilised embryo to the uterus.

**CANCER**: Emotional, moody fallopian tubes which can malfunction during times of high volatility, but on the whole orientated to nurturing travellers in moist environs.

**LEO**: Mercury in a fire sign indicates that the fallopian tubes are vulnerable to ectopic pregnancies – I am not sure if this is a sign of 'stubborness' on the part of the tubes not moving in a proper motion to bring the embryo down into the uterus or if the tube 'thinks' it is the destination point. Mercury in a fire sign indicates inflammations due to all sorts of things, such as infection, fibroids, or just an ectopic pregnancy, and the inflammation caused by that.

**VIRGO**: Mercury-ruled tubes are mostly in good condition, unless otherwise aspected.

**LIBRA**: Unless Venus is in particularly bad shape, the tubes ruled by Libra are good, being an air sign, with no predisposition of ectopic pregnancies or infections.

**SCORPIO**: Sometimes when Mercury is in Scorpio, the tubes can be 'stubborn' and difficulty with peristaltic movement can inhibit the transfer of the embryo to the uterus.

**SAGITTARIUS**: Adventurous fallopian tubes! If one is blocked the other will travel to the other side to pick up an egg from the opposite ovary. Operating always out of the mainstream as Mercury is in detriment in Sagittarius, and therefore beyond expectation, surprise conceptions in spite of physical obstacles are quite normal for these types. Being a fire sign indicates an above average chance of ectopic pregnancy, especially if combust the Sun.

**CAPRICORN**: Conservative thinking equals moderate lifestyle equals fallopian tubes generally in good condition. There is a general feeling of 'stinginess' about Capricorn. At worst, the tubes can be too narrow or not have enough little hairs to assist the transfer of the newly fertilised embryo, or the tubes could be lacking in enough moisture or mucous membranes to facilitate this very necessary movement into the uterus.

**AQUARIUS**: Unpredictable, highly calibrated to the point of being 'hysterical' and prone to cramps and spasms. Aquarius is also ruled by Saturn which rules the skin, skeleton, teeth, bones, and hair. The fallopian tubes are lined with tiny little hairs which help move the newly fertilised embryo down the tube into the uterus for implantation. With Mercury in Aquarius the tubes may go into spasm, failing to move properly, and the little hairs can be incapacitated with the spasm, and not function at all.

**PISCES**: In Mercury's other place of detriment and exile, this position indicates that fertilisation will happen in 'the other place', i.e. perhaps not in the fallopian tubes, but possibly in a petri dish. There might be too much mucus, or moisture in the tubes, thus impeding movement to the uterus.

## General notes

A condition called endometriosis occurs when uterine tissue grows outside of the uterus in the body cavity; it sometimes envelops the ovary or tubes, or forms fibroids in the uterus preventing implantation and conception from taking place. There are various stages of endometriosis and not all of them will prevent a pregnancy. A possible reason for the upswing in the number of women being diagnosed with this could be a result of the very excellent technology of the scanning equipment these days, which reveals polyps of 2mm in some cases. Women have in the past become pregnant naturally in spite of the presence of polyps even bigger than this, but we are led to believe that the condition is 'on the rise'. Astrologically, the signature to look out for is the Saturn/Pluto hard aspect in Libra, and since endometriosis is linked to PCOS, insulin resistance should be considered at the same time. If the Saturn/Pluto conjunction is angular (and this will be a common signature for many women born during the 80s) then it will be more likely that endometriosis will be more of a factor in their reason for not falling pregnant. If this placement is cadent or not affected by more hard aspects from Mars, then go moderately with your interpretation. Bear in mind that this conjunction is in the 'via combusta' and a certain tension will be felt by the client regarding fertility.

## Saturn

If Saturn is the Almuten of Pregancy in a chart, it is actually a most fortunate thing – because the impact of malefics on pregnancy have been reduced by half according to traditional astrology (not using Uranus, Neptune, or Pluto). Typically infertile signatures, such as Saturn conjunct the Moon or Venus or located in the 5th house, can be reinterpreted if Saturn happens to be the Almuten of Pregnancy. Each of these signatures suddenly renders the prognosis remarkably good in terms of someone's ability to achieve pregnancy. The same applies if Mars is the Almuten – its malefic quality on that person's fertility is diminished. However, *and this is important*, the malefic quality in terms of whatever else is going on in that person's chart, is not diminished!

Saturn ruling the 5th house, the Moon, or in aspect to Venus is not on its own an infertile signature, even if it is not the Almuten of Pregnancy.

Since many of the signatures of Saturn with Moon or Venus are normally bad news for fertility, new technologies now mean that previous negative physical qualities can be reversed, or treated with drugs or surgery. Even fifty years ago, bad manifestations of Moon/Saturn would have meant that the condition of the eggs could not have been observed or treated, and fertility treatment would have been guesswork at best. Today, a woman with PCOS has a really good chance at conceiving with her own eggs given the innovation and development of the ICSI technique in the last ten years.

This is one of the inherent misunderstandings of the practical application of astrology to the modern phenomena of infertility. Astrology was developed over thousands of years by people who had no access to the kind of medical technology that we do today. This has to be taken into account when using astrology to treat infertility. Context is everything. So, when clients ask me questions such as: How many children does my chart say I am going to have? I have to respond with – well if you have been using contraception, and postponing child bearing until after you turned twenty-five years of age, then you may have missed all of your potentially fertile times already, but if you had been born in 329 CE you might have had four children by the time you were twenty-two years of age. Questions like these are not easily answered to a generation of people who genuinely think that it is reasonable to expect the physical body to fall pregnant after the age of forty. What astrology does tell us is whether or not a woman might be challenged at some point in her fertile life – and this point is just that – a point in time, not forever and not all the time. So, a woman might have a Saturn/Moon aspect but that doesn't mean she will never have children, just that she might at some point struggle to achieve pregnancy or a live birth. Nowadays physical challenges (such as bad morphology of sperm or eggs that need ICSI) that would have prohibited pregnancy altogether are merely conditions that can be treated.

Saturn also functions as the harbinger of legal responsibilities and duties as citizens of a country or location, which means that with birth comes the inevitable registration of the child born – naming and claiming of parenthood, especially that of the father, and naturally the mother. This birth certificate is a hugely important piece of paper, carrying with it the legal right and entitlement to legacy, property, name from one of the parents, as well as the potential shame of a neglected heritage and reputation, too. So it isn't surprising that Saturn has domicile over the 1st and the 8th houses. Saturn is present in the form of a legal document at your birth and your death – your checking in and checking out of the physical world.

Saturn is also the midwife. It's the last of the seven traditional planets that is visible to the unaided, naked eye. This physical standoff between Saturn, which is visible to earth, and the next planet, the sky god Uranus, is a further representation of the role of Saturn as midwife. Saturn is the boundary between us and the beyond. Saturn chooses who comes in or goes out, much like the hard outer lining of eggs which need ICSI, and the singular sperm making it into the egg, thus eliminating the fertility chances of the other few million sperm.

Saturn is right at the face of reproduction.

So, astrologically in fertility charts, a certain amount of Saturn, in terms of transits to planets, angles or midpoints, is in fact a necessity – not necessarily a limitation. Saturn transits to a natal Moon can be extremely fertile; it seems to underscore the native's possible feelings of impending responsibility with the birth of a child and could hint at the potential for post-natal depression. Falling pregnant and having babies isn't easy, and this transit could be descriptive of the emotional journey the prospective mother is about to embark on, not the denial of a conception per se. Most astrologers will not find it unusual that their clients have babies, marry, and buy or sell property with transits of Saturn to luminaries or angles. This is fairly common, and especially common with a Saturn return.

Again, generationally, the average age of my clients at the moment – and the times in which we live – all point to the very relevant firdaria period of age forty plus in a diurnal chart. I use the nodal firdaria and differentiate between nocturnal and diurnal charts, and at age forty all diurnal charts approach the Saturn firdaria period. As a further annotation to the times in which we, as a collective, live and are having children, it should be mentioned again that the likelihood of a diurnal chart has increased dramatically since the mid-sixties with the increase in caesarean births, which are performed mostly during daylight (business) hours. So we have a large proportion of the population all trying to have children in their Saturn firdaria. So for those clients trying at the age of forty plus, Saturn plays a not insignificant role. Not always for the good, but also not always for the bad.

## A Final Note on Outer Planets

Any malevolent planet in the 1st house is an indicator of something wrong, most probably physical, in the uterus. Physical problems can range from slight to severe, depending on other aspects. An incompetent cervix is easily repaired with a stitch, a fibroid can be removed from the uterus, the lining of the uterus can be increased with medication and acupuncture, and the spontaneous contractions of a 'nervous' uterus can be managed with medication.

Recent chart histories show that with Uranus in Libra (that is, the current generation trying to conceive) and/or where Uranus is in the 1st house (the uterus), surgery to the reproductive organs is likely. Libra rules the reproductive organs in traditional astrology, so it is not unusual to see that women with this placement have often reported surgery for endometriosis (this generation also has Pluto in Libra), or surgery due to other issues. Women with this marker should be checked if they experience miscarriages at around sixteen weeks with no other indicators. For those with Pluto in Libra, PCOS syndrome or endometriosis has now become the most common diagnosis of infertility. For the previous generation of the mid-sixties (with Pluto in Virgo ruled by Mercury), infertility was often diagnosed as a fallopian tube issue. Endometriosis has become 'more common' not because it is really more prevalent, but thanks to advances in medical scanning and technology, smaller polyps (2mm) are being spotted with more frequency. These can be removed using laparoscopic surgery, which is uncomplicated but serves to have an immense placebo effect – the woman now feels that the (bad) reason why she is not falling pregnant has been identified and removed, so the path to parenthood is clear.

A far greater complication is Neptune in the 1st house. Hormonal issues are typically harder to fine-tune, and autoimmune issues are prevalent with this signature. Furthermore, the presence of Neptune here also means that it will be difficult to diagnose, typically needing a second opinion or test; the range of tests is long and detailed so clients are often desperate because the problem is still unclear after so many investigations. Thyroid issues can be common with Neptune in the 1st, but more typically present with aspects between Neptune and the Moon or Venus; moreover if either are in Taurus and configured with Neptune, you can be confident that the endocrine system is somewhat dysfunctional.

## Conclusion

Again, I cannot stress enough that the previous signatures serve as general guides to what I have found in my nearly two decades of practice and research. Always make sure to engage your client individually and employ active listening to receive their story. Examine the charts carefully in light of that, and make your judgements in the light of everything you've learned and what the astrology shows you. With the rapid developments in the fertility industry and reproductive science, we have to stay vigilant in our astrological reasoning and allow for new insights to inform ancient wisdom. And above all else, make sure to do no harm.

## Notes

96. Barbara Tedlock, 'Seeing With Different Eyes: The Diviner's Space Time', *The Journal of Shamanic Practices* 2.2 (2009): pp.5–9.
97. See *Liber Hermetis*.
98. *A Handbook of Medical Astrology*.
99. Ibid.
100. http://www.dailymail.co.uk/health/article-153278/Viagra-boosts-fertility-hopes.html
101. Aristotle and Barnes, J. *Complete Works of Aristotle, Volume 2: The Revised Oxford Translation*.
102. *A Handbook of Medical Astrology*, p.83.
103. http://www.medic8.com/healthguide/articles/prolactin.html
104. *Infertility: A Sympathetic Approach*, p.141.
105. Cf., Winston on lifestyle changes affecting sperm quality, cited above.
106. *A Handbook of Medical Astrology*, p.52.
107. Ibid.
108. Ibid.
109. Brady, Bernadette. *Medieval Astrology Certificate Study Guide*.
110. *A Handbook of Medical Astrology*.
111. Ibid.

# 9

# A Concluding Parable

The Astronomer bowed… 'Her-Bak, look west… now turn slowly to the east, watching the sky. What do you see?'
'As I turn I keep on seeing new stars'.
'If you stand still all night what will you see?'
'I shall see the stars passing before me'.
'What moves? The stars or yourself watching them?'
'If I stand still it must be the stars that move'. Her-Bak paused.
'Unless Earth turns as I have just done. Is this possible?'
The Astronomer smiled at his bewilderment. He gave the disciple time to think, then asked, 'If the stars move, if Sun and Moon travel, why should Earth alone in the cosmos stand still? The idea repels you?'
'It would be strange', Her-Bak replied, 'if one had to imagine that Earth, that seemed still in the shifting sky, was on the move. But everything I learn proves that my senses are subject to illusion… I don't dare deny that such movement takes place if you tell me it is so'.
The Astronomer watched Her-Bak benevolently. 'I will make no statement', he said. 'Your experience of illusion is enough to make you careful. What matters to Earth's inhabitants is that they should know of their vital connection with the sky. As to the movement of the stars, it is better to note what you see than to imagine what may deflect you from the real meaning. Then we will place ourselves at the center of the sky we are watching, where all star-movement is seen by reference to ourselves'.[112]

In this parable, Isha Schwaller de Lubicz hints at how we should approach the mythological sky. She suggests that geocentrism is not a way of emphasising our importance in the cosmos; rather, from a Platonic perspective, by placing ourselves at the centre of the universe we make ourselves subject to the influences from the heavenly realms. The stars, and the narratives they carry, have particular meaning to the person standing on earth observing them, wherever that might be, whatever cultural perspective they adopt. We place ourselves in the narrative, we connect to the sky.

The myths that have been passed down through the ages are a collection of these stories from various perspectives around the world; most narratives are similar, some present differences in terms of detail, but not plot. The ultimate question when encountering or experiencing a myth is; 'what does this mean to and for me?' Implicit in this question is that once meaning is ascertained, action is required – sometimes with the help of an astrologer or a psychodynamic therapist. Little value is to be gained through literal interpretation; the real turning point is the realisation that the myth contains a personal message for the observer. Living in the paradox of knowing the illusion and finding a truth in it is key to a creative life.

Myths are dead until they are taken up. They speak to us once we recognise ourselves in them, through a dialogue. As practising astrologers, we can recognise the myths that appear to be active in the client's lived experience, and by retelling the story of the myth through the language of astrology, we guide the client to understanding. As I hope to have shown, astrology also functions through narrative healing and through language and the hermeneutics of symbolism.

There are many meanings and many layers, yet only one opportunity to resonate with the client. In the emotionally-charged field of fertility astrology, we have an enormous responsibility: our clients not only look to us for practical guidance, but also rely on us to help them navigate the arduous but extraordinary journey towards their own healing.

**Notes**

112. Schwaller de Lubicz, Isha. *Her-Bak: The Living Face of Ancient Egypt*.

# Appendix

## Almuten Worksheet

| POINT ON CHART | ☉ | ☿ | ☽ | ♀ | ♂ | ♃ | ♄ |
|---|---|---|---|---|---|---|---|
| ASC | | | | | | | |
| | | | | | | | |
| RULER OF ASC | | | | | | | |
| | | | | | | | |
| MOON | | | | | | | |
| | | | | | | | |
| RULER OF MOON | | | | | | | |
| | | | | | | | |
| 5TH CUSP | | | | | | | |
| | | | | | | | |
| RULER OF 5TH | | | | | | | |
| | | | | | | | |
| POSITION JUP | | | | | | | |
| | | | | | | | |
| PLANETS IN 5TH | | | | | | | |
| | | | | | | | |
| TOTALS | | | | | | | |

# Glossary

**Alcocoden also Alcocodon, Alchocoden**
Also known to Perso-Arabic authors as kadhkhudāh or al-kadhudāh. The planet that holds rulership over the degree of the planet or place taken as hyleg ('giver or life'), whilst bearing an aspect to the hyleg. It was used as the 'giver of years' since its general nature and fortitude was used to define the natural years of a life. See http://www.skyscript.co.uk/gl/alchocoden.html

**Almuten**
The strongest planet when all essential dignities are considered. The term is Arabic and derives from al-mateen, meaning 'the firm one' or 'strong in power', but the concept exists in the works of Ptolemy and other early classical astrologers. The method of identifying the almuten involves considering the full range of essential dignities, so that rulership by sign, exaltation, triplicity, term and face is considered – not just rulership by sign. Hence Venus is said to rule the sign of Libra but Saturn is the almuten, being capable of assuming rulership by exaltation, triplicity, term and face.

A point-scoring technique is often used to determine the almuten of any given point. This, and further details are outlined in part 5 of the tutorial 'Understanding Planetary Dignity and Debility'. See http://www.skyscript.co.uk/gl/almuten.html

**Artificial Insemination**
The general name for the procedure in which sperm are inserted directly into a woman's cervix, fallopian tubes, or uterus.

**Blastocyst**
This stage of embryo development is achieved around 5 days after the egg is fertilized.

### Combustion/combust
A planet is combust when it is in conjunction with the Sun and therefore hidden from sight by the light of the Sun. Traditionally this is a serious debility and implies that the planet is weakened or restricted in power. However, if the planet is within 17 minutes of the Sun, it is termed Cazimi – in the heart of the Sun – and considered strengthened by the union. See http://www.skyscript.co.uk/gl/combust.html

### Dysmenorrhea/Amenorrhea
A condition in which a woman doesn't have menstrual periods.

### Ectopic Pregnancy
When an embryo implants outside the uterus.

### Endometriosis
A painful condition in which tissue from the lining of the uterus (the endometrium) grows outside of the uterus.

### Egg Retrieval
The procedure during an IVF cycle where the oocytes (eggs) are harvested through a minimally-invasive surgical procedure. This is done under light anesthesia so that patients are sleeping during the entire process. Typically takes about 30 minutes from start to finish.

### Embryo
The term used to describe the early stages of fetal growth. Strictly defined from the second to the ninth week of pregnancy but often used to designate any time after conception.

### Embryo Transfer
The procedure of transferring embryos back in to the endometrial cavity (womb) of a patient during an IVF cycle. It occurs on the third or fifth day after an egg retrieval.

### Follicle Stimulating Hormone (FSH)
A hormone produced in the pituitary gland that causes cells in the ovaries to grow. Sold under the names Follistim, Fertinex, and Gonal-F.

**Fibroids**
Overgrowth of the muscular tissue of the uterus. Fibroids are typically knotty masses of benign muscle tissue that can distort the shape and function of the uterus. They are typically classified into three categories: sub-mucosal, intramural and sub-serosal. Sub-mucosal fibroids are found in the uterine cavity and impair implantation. They need to be removed in order to conceive. Intramural fibroids are problematic when they become severely enlarged or impinge on the uterine cavity. Sub-serosal fibroids are generally left alone during fertility treatments.

**Follicle**
A fluid-filled pocket in the ovary that houses the microscopic egg. Each ovary has many follicles within it. Follicles start out extremely small and then grow larger under the influence of hormones (and the medications that mimic these hormones). Follicles are lined with granulosa cells which produce estrogen and nourish the oocyte (egg). Each follicle contains a single oocyte.

**Gamete Intrafallopian Transfer (GIFT)**
An assisted reproductive technique that involves removing sperm and eggs, mixing them together and placing them into the fallopian tubes.

**Heliacal rising/setting**
Ancient astrologers gave particular emphasis to the heliacal rising and setting of stars since these could be used as reliable indicators to agricultural conditions. A heliacal setting occurs when a planet or star enters into conjunction with the Sun. The increasing proximity of the Sun towards the star each day eventually leads to a period of invisibility, during which it is masked by the Sun's light (see 'combust'). Its setting is the moment when it is visible for the last time immediately after sunset. It then rises and sets with the Sun, remaining hidden from sight both day and night. When the Sun has separated from the star by somewhere between 8-20 degrees of zodiacal longitude the star begins to emerge, briefly, immediately before sunrise – its first brief appearance being known as its heliacal rising.

### Hyleg

Also known as Hayláj, Hylech, Apheta, Alpheta or 'Prorogator of Life'. The planet or point considered to have the greatest influence upon vitality and so known as 'the giver of life'. It was used in the calculation of the length of life, and directions or contacts between the hyleg and destructive planets or places (Anareta) were used to mark periods where life was endangered. The strength and fortitude of the ruler of the Hyleg, the Alchocoden, was also considered.

An 'hylegiacal' or 'aphetic' place relates to the houses in which Ptolemy claimed that any planet to be admitted as hyleg must be located. These are (in order of preference): - the 1st, 10th, 11th, 7th or 9th houses.

Ptolemy stated that only the Sun, Moon, Ascendant, Midheaven or Part of Fortune could be admitted as hyleg, but later astrologers also allowed Venus and Jupiter or a planet that dominated the pre-natal lunation. See http://www.skyscript.co.uk/gl/hyleg.html

### Intracytoplasmic Sperm Injection (ICSI)

Placement of a single sperm into a single oocyte (egg) by penetrating the outer coatings of the egg. This technique is used in cases where there are very low sperm numbers, motility or morphology. ICSI is also used for patients who have had previous IVF cycles with failed fertilization.

### Intra-Uterine Insemination (IUI)

A technique that transfers sperm directly in to the uterus. It bypasses the vaginal and cervical defense mechanisms of the female reproductive tract and allows better sperm delivery to the fallopian tubes. This allows the sperm and egg to interact in close proximity. It is a very common treatment for mild and moderate deficits in the semen analysis. IUI is typically used in conjunction with medications that increase the number of eggs per cycle and triggering of ovulation. The goal is to have more 'targets' for the sperm (eggs), perfect timing and better sperm delivery.

### In Vitro Fertilization (IVF)

A powerful procedure to help patients conceive pregnancies. IVF entails stimulating your ovaries to develop multiple follicles. This is achieved with injectable medications. The goal of IVF is to produce a large number of growing follicles, then harvest the eggs inside the follicles through a short surgical procedure performed in the doctor's office. The eggs are then inseminated with sperm in the laboratory, sometimes using ICSI, in order to create embryos that can then be transferred back to the endometrial cavity (the womb) of the patient. The name in vitro fertilization refers to the fact that the oocyte is fertilized by the sperm in the laboratory, rather than inside the female reproductive tract.

**Joy**
The house where each of the traditional planets is assumed to be especially strong: Moon – 3rd house; Mercury – 1st house; Venus – 5th house; Sun – 9th house; Mars – 6th house; Jupiter – 11th house; Saturn – 12th house.

**Katarche/ic**
The word 'katarche' is often interpreted as 'beginning' or 'inception' but we get a much better sense of its meaning in ancient astrology by the alternative rendering 'auguration' or 'inauguration'. This word is usually used today to describe a ceremonial beginning or formal commencement (such as a formal induction into office). However, it also originates from the word 'augur' which developed into the related Latin words auspice and augury. See http://www.skyscript.co.uk/gl/katarche.html

**Laparoscopic/laparoscopy**
A procedure that involves the insertion of a narrow, telescope-like instrument called a laparoscope through a small incision in the abdomen; this used to perform surgery to the fallopian tubes in fertility patients, but also for other abdominal surgeries.

**LGBTQI+**
Umbrella acronym for Lesbian, Gay, Bisexual, Trans and Queer people.

**Morphology/motility**
Morphology: The size and shape of sperm.
Motility: The ability of sperm to move by themselves.

**Oligospermia**
When a man has too few sperm to fertilize an egg normally.

### Paran/s or paranatellonta

Paranatellonta are stars or star groups that fall upon angles at the same time that a significant constellation or planet is also upon the angles. They are viewed as attendants. In ancient astrology the term was also applied to the constellations that ascended with the zodiacal decans.

In modern astrology the term Paran (short for Paranatellonta) is generally used to describe stars or planets that are angular as a planet hits the Ascendant, MC, Descendant or IC. For example, the parans of Mercury would be those stars or planets that were rising, culminating, descending or located upon the IC at the same time that Mercury is in any or those positions. Thus if the fixed star Regulus culminates on the Midheaven as Mercury rises on the Ascendant it is referred to as a paran of Mercury and considered to have an influence upon the planet's meaning. See http://www.skyscript.co.uk/gl/paran.html

### Polycystic Ovary Syndrome (PCOS)

A common hormonal condition in which an imbalance in the sex hormones may cause menstrual abnormalities, skin and hair changes, obesity, infertility and other long-term health problems. The name comes from the multiple small cysts which line the ovaries of most women with the disorder.

### Preimplantation Genetic Diagnosis (PGD)

A technique for identifying genetic or chromosomal information about embryos before transferring them back to a patient's endometrial cavity (the womb). It entails taking a biopsy of the embryo on day three after egg retrieval. PGD can be employed to identify embryos that carry a genetic disease that may be asymptomatically carried by the parents, or it may be used to identify explanations for Recurrent Pregnancy Loss and improve pregnancy outcomes in selected patients.

### Varicocele

A varicose vein in the scrotum that may affect the quality and production of sperm.

# Bibliography

Aristotle and Barnes, J. *Complete Works of Aristotle, Volume 2: The Revised Oxford Translation*. 6th edition. Ed. Jonathan Barnes. (Princeton N.J.: Princeton University Press, 1984.)

Bonatti, Guido. *The Book of Astronomy*. Trans. Benjamin Dykes. (Minneapolis, MA: Cazimi Press, 2007.)

Brady, Bernadette. *Medieval Astrology Certificate Study Guide*. (Bristol, England: Astro Logos, 1999–2003.)

———, *Starlight: Returning the Stars to Astrology*, Version 1.0 (Barneswood Ltd, 2002).

———, *Brady's Book of Fixed Stars* (York Beach, Maine: Samuel Weiser Inc, 1998, pp.84-85.)

Campion, Nicholas. *The Dawn of Astrology: A Cultural History of Western Astrology – The Ancient and Classical Worlds*. (London: Hambledon Continuum, 2008.)

Charon, Rita. *Narrative Medicine: Honoring the stories of illness*. (New York: Oxford University Press, 2008.)

Cornelius, Geoffrey. *The Moment of Astrology*. 2nd edition. (Bournemouth, England: The Wessex Astrologer Ltd, 2002.)

Dorotheus of Sidon, *Carmen Astrologicum*. Trans. David Pingree. (Mansfield, England: Ascella, 1993.)

Dykes, B. *Introduction to Traditional Astrology: Abu Ma'shar and al-Qabisi*. (Minneapolis, MN: Cazimi Press, 2011.)

Ebertin, Reinhold. *The Combination of Stellar Influences (COSI)*. (Tempe, AZ: AFA, 1972.)

Elder, Kay, Baker, Doris J., and Ribes, Julie A. *Infections, Infertility, and Assisted Reproduction*. (Cambridge, England: Cambridge University Press, 2005, p.7.)

Foucault, M. and Hurley, R. *The History of Sexuality: The Use of Pleasure, Vol. 2*. (New York: Knopf Doubleday Publishing Group, 1990.)

_____, *The History of Sexuality: The Care of the Self, Vol. 3*. (New York: Knopf Doubleday Publishing Group, 1990.)

Gainsburg, Adam. *The Light of Venus*. (Burke, VA: Soulsign, 2012.)

Goldacre, Ben. *Bad Science*. (London: Fourth Estate, 2008.)

Greene, Liz. *Saturn: A New Look at an Old Devil*. (Wellingborough, England: Aquarian Press, 1983.)

Gunzburg, Darrelyn. 'How Do Astrologers Read Charts?', *Astrologies: Plurality and Diversity*. (Ceredigion, Wales: Sophia Centre Press, 2013.)

Hartouni, Valerie. *Cultural Conceptions*. (Minneapolis: University of Minnesota Press, 1997.)

Hermes Trismegistus, *Liber Hermetis*. Trans. Robert Zoller, ed. Robert Hand. (Spica, 1998. 1st ed.1993. Project Hindsight.)

Jobes, Gertrude and James. *Outer Space: Myths, Name Meanings, Calendars*. (New York: Scarecrow Press, 1964, p.126.)

Kirsch, I. *The Emperor's New Drugs: Exploding the Antidepressant Myth*. (London: The Bodley Head. 2009.)

Mattingly, C. *The Paradox of Hope: Journeys Through a Clinical Borderland*. (Berkeley: University of California Press, 2010.)

Moerman, D.E. and Jonas, W.B. 'Deconstructing the Placebo Effect and Finding the Meaning Response.' *Annals of Internal Medicine*. (Philadelphia, PA: American College of Physicians, 136, pp.471-476, 2002.)

Nauman, Eileen. *Medical Astrology*, 3rd. edition. (Cottonwood, AZ: Blue Turtle Publishing, 1996, p.36.)

Omar of Tiberias, *Three Books on Nativities*. Ed. Robert Schmidt, trans. Robert Hand, vol. xiv. (Berkeley Springs, VA: The Golden Hind Press, Project Hindsight, 1997.)

Ostrander, Sheila and Schroeder, Lynn. *Astrological Birth Control*. (Englewood Cliffs, NJ: Prentice-Hall, 1972.)

Perera, Silvia Brinton. *Descent to the Goddess: A Way of Initiation for Women*. (Toronto: Inner City Books, 1981.)

Ridder-Patrick, Jane. *A Handbook of Medical Astrology*. (Contemporary Astrology Series. New York: Arkana, 1990.)

_____, *A Handbook of Medical Astrology*, 2nd edition. (Edinburgh: CrabApple Press, 2007, p.76.)

_____, 'The Healing Power of Astrology', (*The Astrological Journal*, July/August 2014: pp.11–15.)

Schwaller de Lubicz, Isha. *Her-Bak: The Living Face of Ancient Egypt*. (Rochester, VT: Inner Traditions, 1978.)

Shaw, Gregory. 'The Chora of the Timaeus and Iamblichean Theurgy.' (*Horizons* pp.103-129, vol.3, no.2, 2012.)

Tedlock, Barbara. 'Seeing With Different Eyes: The Diviner's Space Time', (*The Journal of Shamanic Practices* 2.2, 2009: pp.5–9.)

Winston, Prof. Robert. *Infertility: A Sympathetic Approach to Understanding the Causes and Treatment*. (London: Edbury Digital, 2013.) https://www.penguin.co.uk/books/1019605/infertility/

Wolkenstein, Diane, and Kramer, Samuel Noah. *Inanna: Queen of Heaven and Earth*. (New York: Harper & Row, 1983.)

_____, *Sumerian Mythology* (Philadelphia: University of Pennsylvania Press, 1961)

# Other Titles from The Wessex Astrologer
## www.wessexastrologer.com

*Martin Davis*
Astrolocality Astrology: A Guide to What it is and How to Use it
From Here to There: An Astrologer's Guide to Astromapping

*Wanda Sellar*
The Consultation Chart
An Introduction to Medical Astrology
An Introduction to Decumbiture

*Geoffrey Cornelius*
The Moment of Astrology

*Darrelyn Gunzburg*
Life After Grief: An Astrological Guide to Dealing with Grief
AstroGraphology: The Hidden Link between your Horoscope and your Handwriting

*Paul F. Newman*
Declination: The Steps of the Sun
Luna: The Book of the Moon

*Deborah Houlding*
The Houses: Temples of the Sky

*Dorian Geiseler Greenbaum*
Temperament: Astrology's Forgotten Key

*Howard Sasportas*
The Gods of Change

*Patricia L. Walsh*
Understanding Karmic Complexes

*M. Kelly Hunter*
Living Lilith: the Four Dimensions of the Cosmic Feminine

*Barbara Dunn*
Horary Astrology Re-Examined

*Deva Green*
Evolutionary Astrology

*Jeff Green*
Pluto Volume 1: The Evolutionary Journey of the Soul
Pluto Volume 2: The Evolutionary Journey of the Soul Through Relationships
Essays on Evolutionary Astrology (ed. by Deva Green)

*Dolores Ashcroft-Nowicki and Stephanie V. Norris*
The Door Unlocked: An Astrological Insight into Initiation

*Greg Bogart*
Astrology and Meditation: The Fearless Contemplation of Change

*Henry Seltzer*
The Tenth Planet: Revelations from the Astrological Eris

*Ray Grasse*
Under a Sacred Sky: Essays on the Practice and Philosophy of Astrology

*Martin Gansten*
**Primary Directions**

*Joseph Crane*
Astrological Roots: The Hellenistic Legacy
Between Fortune and Providence

*Bruce Scofield*
Day-Signs: Native American Astrology from Ancient Mexico

*Komilla Sutton*
The Essentials of Vedic Astrology
The Lunar Nodes: Crisis and Redemption
Personal Panchanga: The Five Sources of Light
The Nakshatras: the Stars Beyond the Zodiac

*Anthony Louis*
The Art of Forecasting using Solar Returns

*Oscar Hofman*
Classical Medical Astrology

*Bernadette Brady*
Astrology, A Place in Chaos
Star and Planet Combinations

*Richard Idemon*
The Magic Thread
Through the Looking Glass

*Nick Campion*
The Book of World Horoscopes

*Judy Hall*
Patterns of the Past
Karmic Connections
Good Vibrations
The Soulmate Myth: A Dream Come True or Your Worst Nightmare?
The Book of Why: Understanding your Soul's Journey
Book of Psychic Development

*Neil D. Paris*
Surfing your Solar Cycles

*Michele Finey*
The Sacred Dance of Venus and Mars

*David Hamblin*
The Spirit of Numbers

*Dennis Elwell*
Cosmic Loom

*Bob Makransky*
Planetary Strength
Planetary Hours
Planetary Combination

*Petros Eleftheriadis*
Horary Astrology: The Practical Guide to Your Fate